Aesthetic Surgery of the Craniofacial Skeleton

Springer Science+Business Media, LLC

With a Foreword by Fernando Ortiz Monasterio, M.D.

With Illustrations by Min Li, M.D., and Li-Jun Zhao, B.F.A.

With Contributions by

Joseph G. McCarthy, M.D.
Lawrence D. Bell Professor of Plastic Surgery
Director, Institute of Reconstructive Plastic Surgery
New York University Medical Center

Barry L. Eppley, M.D., D.M.D.
Assistant Professor of Surgery
Section of Plastic Surgery
Indiana University Medical Center

Robert J. Havlik, M.D.
Assistant Professor of Surgery
Section of Plastic Surgery
Indiana University Medical Center

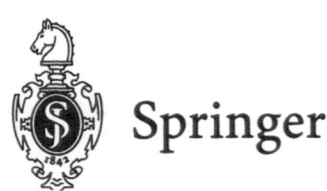 Springer

Min Li, M.D., M.S., M.F.A.
Attending Plastic Surgeon
Medical Illustrator and Sculptor
People's Republic of China

John J. Coleman III, M.D.
Professor of Surgery
Chairman, Section of Plastic
  Surgery
Indiana University Medical Center

A. Michael Sadove, M.D.
Professor of Surgery
Director of Craniofacial Program
Indiana University Medical Center

Aesthetic Surgery of the Craniofacial Skeleton

An Atlas

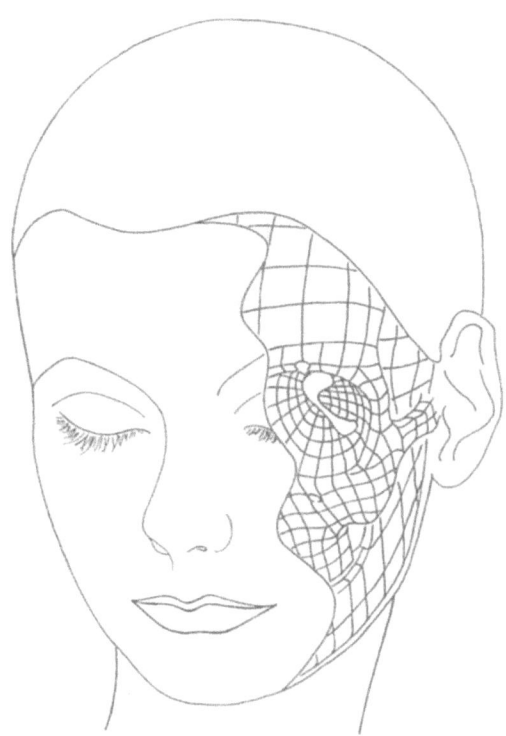

Min Li, M.D., M.S., M.F.A.
Department of Surgery, Section of
  Plastic Surgery
Indiana University Medical Center
Emerson Hall 235
545 Barnhill Drive
Indianapolis, IN 46202-5124, USA

John J. Coleman, III, M.D.
Department of Surgery, Section of
  Plastic Surgery
Indiana University Medical Center
Emerson Hall 235
545 Barnhill Drive
Indianapolis, IN 46202-5124, USA

A. Michael Sadove, M.D.
Department of Surgery, Section of
  Plastic Surgery
Indiana University Medical Center
Emerson Hall 235
545 Barnhill Drive
Indianapolis, IN 46202-5124, USA

Cover design and illustration labeling: Gary Schmitt

Library of Congress Cataloging-in-Publication Data
Li, Min, M.D.
   Aesthetic surgery of the craniofacial skeleton : an atlas / Min Li, John J. Coleman
III, A. Michael Sadove; foreword by Fernando Ortiz Monasterio ;
illustrations by Min Li and Li-Jun Zhao ; contribution by Barry L.
Eppley, Robert J. Havlik.
     p.   cm.
  Includes bibliographical references and index.
   ISBN 978-1-4612-7344-8   ISBN 978-1-4612-1930-9 (eBook)
   DOI 10.1007/978-1-4612-1930-9
   1. Face—Surgery. 2. Skull—Surgery. 3. Surgery, Plastic.
I. Coleman, John J., 1947-   . II. Sadove, A. Michael. III. Title.
   [DNLM: 1. Facial Bones—surgery—atlases. 2. Skull—surgery—
atlases. 3. Surgery, Plastic—methods—atlases. 4. Osteotomy—
methods—atlases. WE 17 L693a 1996]
RD119.5.F33L5 1996
617.5'20592—dc20   96-13192

Printed on acid-free paper.

Production coordinated by Chernow Editorial Services, Inc., and managed by Karen
Phillips; manufacturing supervised by Rhea Talbert.
Typeset by Bytheway Typesetting Services, Inc., Norwich, NY.

9 8 7 6 5 4 3 2 1

ISBN 978-1-4612-7344-8

To our parents and teachers,
who made the opportunities possible

Foreword

Surgery of the facial skeleton has been performed for many years for the treatment of tumors and for the repair of facial fractures. Considerable advancements were made during the First World War, and by the Second World War, maxillofacial surgery was a well-established field. Early this century, daring surgeons used many of the osteotomies we now use electively for aesthetic surgery as an approach to tumors deeply located in the face. The outstanding contributions of Paul Tessier extended the field of maxillofacial surgery into the orbit and the cranium, converting the relatively limited field of maxillofacial surgery into a more complex speciality and making possible the correction of major deformities considered impossible before.

Similar to the early attempts to cut the facial bones in order to reach deeper structures, the new advances in craniofacial surgery permit us to reach inside the cranial base at the junction of the facial bones and the cranial face and remove tumors previously considered unreachable. The benefits of these advancements extended to the field of trauma, allowing more accurate reconstructions, improved rigid fixation, and bone grafting at the acute stage reducing to a minimum the sequelae of the injury.

Following the work of Tessier, considerable experience has accumulated in the treatment of tumors, congenital deformities, and trauma. Complications have been reduced to a minimum and results are predictable. Outstanding advances in imaging instrumentation, and other technical aids have decreased operating time, thus converting some of this very major surgery into an everyday practice.

As a result of this progress, many of these procedures performed on the craniofacial skeleton have now been incorporated into the practice of aesthetic surgery performed electively to improve facial contour and harmony. Although the field of aesthetic surgery of the craniofacial skeleton includes many long-accepted soft tissue procedures, as well as alterations of ligament and muscle insertions, the authors have chosen to present in this book a synthetic general prospectus of the osteotomies around the craniofacial skeleton.

This *Aesthetic Surgery of the Craniofacial Skeleton* presents the basic approach of incisions, instrumentation, bone graft harvest, and osteotomies that the readers interested in this type of surgery will find useful.

FERNANDO ORTIZ MONASTERIO, M.D.

Preface

Craniofacial surgery began as an expansion and refinement of the surgical techniques and approaches of maxillofacial plastic surgery. Paul Tessier's bold approach to movement of large blocks of the calvarium, their attached facial skeleton and the subsequent confirmation of his contention that bone grafts would provide the stability necessary to maintain these manipulations, revolutionized the surgical approach to severe congenital anomalies of the head and face. That these maneuvers could be effected through incisions in the oral cavity, behind the hairline and within the orbit, fostered the notion that the radical skull manipulation of the face necessary to improve the life of deformed children could also be extended to the purview of cosmetic surgery. So as with many other techniques in plastic surgery (skin grafting, microsurgery, etc.), the initial application to severe problems of life-threatening nature has been extended to problems less desperate, but still of importance, in fact, to elective surgery and aesthetic surgery. In the last ten years, the refinement of analysis by life-size photography and cephalometric measurements, the improvement in instrumentation and operative technique, and the critical evaluation of results, have made craniofacial aesthetic surgery a reality. Frustration with results of surgery that addresses only facial soft tissue and specific requests from a more knowledgeable consumer have led to the acceptance of osteotomy and bone movement as an integral part of aesthetic surgery.

Crucial to the understanding of aesthetic surgery and to the extension into the craniofacial arena is the fact that most aesthetic procedures are performed on what is basically a "normal craniofacial skeleton." Thus, the attempt to improve appearance must address normal anatomy and the manipulation must create a result deemed more desirable by the patient and acceptable to the surgeon. Beauty itself is an uncertain concept, depending upon human emotion. The face is a three dimensional structure with innumerable changing shapes. To define an absolute set of parameters that constitute beauty, even within a single culture, is impossible in this fluid medium. Yet the skeleton of the face provides the most static componet of this difficult milieu and the one which can be changed and subsequently measured most precisely. Thus, aesthetic craniofacial surgery may allow more accurate assessment of success and failure in this very subjective endeavor.

This text attempts to be a comprehensive exposition of the osteotomies used in aesthetic craniofacial surgery. Each technique is presented in diagrammatic form with the instruments appropriate for its execution. An encyclopedic approach to the problem means inclusion of detailed drawings and text on instruments used. Patient preparation and positioning for surgery is also discussed. Drawings of the preoperative deformity with and without soft tissue, the osteotomy and the desired postoperative result will hopefully provide a realistic schema of presently accepted technique in a framework upon which practitioners can extend these mehtods for the future benefit of the patient. Because facial beauty is a subjective and culturally defined trait, many of the osteotomies described in this text are not commonly used in the practice of plastic surgery in the western world. Although the intent is not to catalog Oriental aesthetic technique, a description of these osteotomies is important in such an inclusive text and should improve our understanding of world-wide aesthetic principles and problems.

What then is the goal of the book? For the initiated, may it be an encyclopedia of technique with detail enough to provide an easily understood approach to the numerous aesthetic manipulations of the skeleton; for the experienced surgeon, a comprehensive exposition of successfully performed procedures which may be applied, adapted or rejected depending on the analysis of his patient's problem; for the patient, the ultimate recipient, a catalyst for improvement in the emerging discipline of aesthetic craniofacial surgery.

MIN LI, M.D., M.S., M.F.A.
JOHN J. COLEMAN III, M.D.
A. MICHAEL SADOVE, M.D.

Acknowledgments

We wish first to express our gratitude to those, especially Fernando Otiz Monasterio, M.D., who wrote the foreword, and to Joseph G. McCarthy, who contributed to the writing of the chapters.

Our special thanks to Ms. Barbara A. Chernow for her expert revision of manuscripts for presentation to the publisher.

A very profound appreciation is given to Ms. Esther Gumpert, and the entire staff of Springer-Verlag for their support, encouragement, and guidance throughout this project.

Our thanks also to the staffs in section of plastic surgery at Indiana University Medical Center.

Finally, we would like to thank our families for their love, support, and understanding. Without any of these people, there obviously would have been no book.

Contents

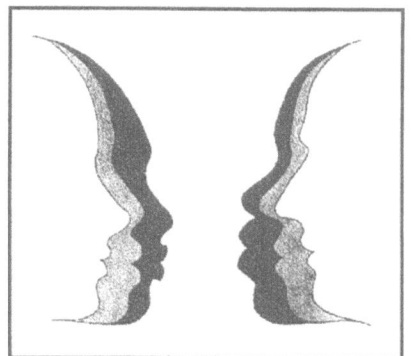

1

Beautiful
Faces

What kind of face is beautiful? This question seems impossible to answer. The answer would certainly depend on the race, sex, and age of the person who is judging and the era in which the person lives. Is there any way to define a beautiful face? Yes. According to aesthetic research, beautiful things generally give rise to pleasing feelings. Likewise, a beautiful face should have character and be attractive and pleasing.

Form and color determine whether an object is beautiful or not. Both form and color possess a series of varying qualities, such as proportion, rhythm, meter, contrast, symmetry, and so on. These qualities combine and constitute all the things we see. Some of the things are beautiful. Others are ordinary or ugly. Any single quality cannot be defined as beauty. The golden proportion is generally considered beautiful, however, if all faces were in this proportion exactly, the world should be a boring and uninteresting place to live.

Although craniofacial surgery will change the color of a face, resulting from stretching of the skin and greater light reflection after augmentation, it depends primarily on changing facial form to shape a beautiful face.

Most descriptions about faces are descriptions in two dimensions. In clinical work, we need to evaluate a face in three dimensions. For example, the distance between the eyes of a person with deep eye sockets may appear to be shorter than that of the average person. Likewise, we will perceive the nose to be a little bit longer after a simple saddle nose correction. All these discrepancies between our perceptions and two-dimensional measurements are three-dimensional effects. Our perception of the shape of an object depends on the volumetric proportion of neighboring objects. So plastic surgeons should train themselves to evaluate faces three dimensionally, not depending solely on two-dimensional measurements.

A face is a complex three-dimensional form. It can be considered to consist of many simpler and smaller geometric forms and the latter can be decomposed into even simpler and even smaller forms (Figure 1-1). The preoperative evaluation and design of aesthetic craniofacial surgery are based on changing the volumes of these smaller geometric forms to affect our perception of the overall facial form. Although, as discussed above, it is impossible to define an absolute boundary for beautiful faces, some general considerations can be suggested. First, a beautiful face should be symmetric from side to side. Secondly, the volume proportions between areas such as forehead, nose, chin, and so on should be proportional and follow a visual rhythm. Last, the transition between regions should be smooth and continuous. All of the volumes form an integral and harmonious unit rather than a simple collection of the different geometric forms. Beautiful faces are like wonderful symphonies. The simple and small geometric forms are the notes of music that combine and interact to form the many beautiful faces.

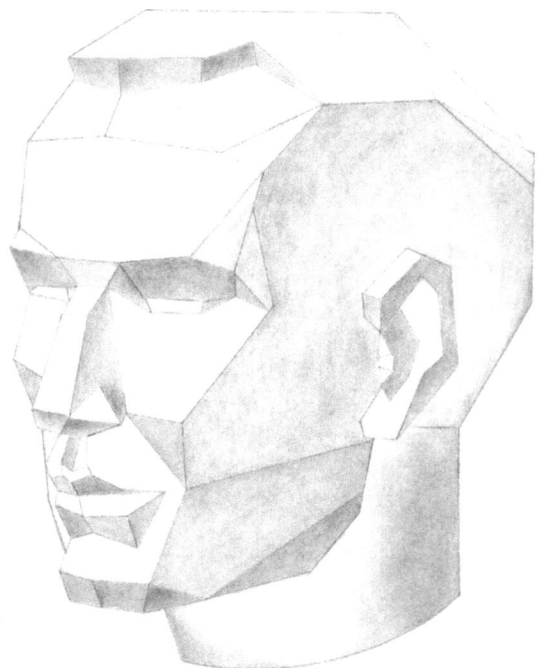

Figure 1-1 A face can be decomposed into several simpler forms.

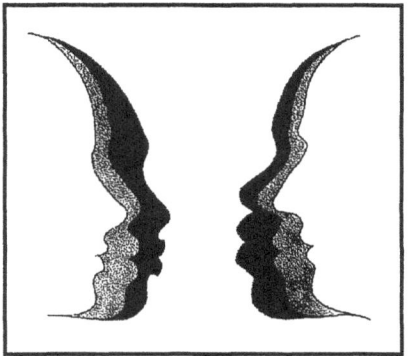

2

Aesthetic Training

An excellent plastic surgeon should possess the qualities of both a surgeon and an artist. Every surgeon has the former, but not all plastic surgeons have the latter. Since plastic surgeons construct beautiful forms, it is very important for them to have good aesthetic judgment and a sense of three-dimensional forms.

Some plastic surgeons have excellent operative skills, but the results of their operations are not beautiful. Plastic surgeons should systematically study aesthetic theory and strive to develop better aesthetic judgments, a sense of shapes, and the ability of spatial imagination.

There are many techniques to develop aesthetic sense, including painting, sculpture, photography, and observation and evaluation. Some suggested exercises follow.

Painting

- Sketch a head accurately. Strive to paint the expression on the face.
- Observe the subject through the caricaturist's eye. Figure out the characteristics and draw them down in the exaggerated and concise strokes.
- Recall a subject you saw a short while ago on television or on the street, and try to draw that person's face.
- Record operations you performed with illustrations.

Sculpture

- Make a clay sculpture of the head of a model.
- Sculpt from a photograph.
- Make a portrait relief from a photograph.
- Make a caricature sculpture.

Photography

- Take black-and-white photos and develop a sense about light and form.

Observation and Evaluation

- We see many different people around us everyday. Study their faces and determine their characteristics. From aesthetic point of view, make some evaluations for possible plastic surgical operations.

After practicing the above-mentioned techniques for a period of time, you will experience marked improvement in aesthetic sense and sense of three-dimensional forms.

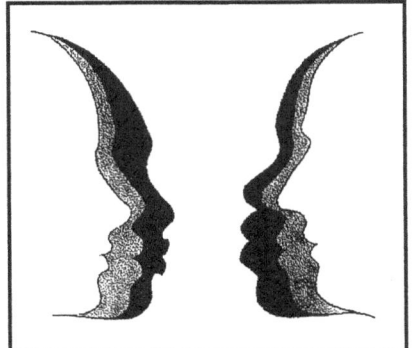

Facial Forms

To reshape facial skeletons, one needs a comprehensive understanding of facial form. This understanding includes quantitative measurements and qualitative perceptions. Anthropometry is the former, which describes the skull, a very irregular three-dimensional object, by measuring the distances between certain points on the skull, calculating the standard deviations of those distances, and presenting the variations of any individual. Anthropometry identifies a range of normality. However, the aim of aesthetic craniofacial surgery is to construct a beautiful, pleasing, and attractive face. It makes a comparison between the preoperation and the postoperation appearances of the same individual, rather than a comparison between the individual and the whole population. In addition, anthropometry describes a skull in numbers. It is hard to imagine three-dimensional forms from a series of numbers.

According to the psychological research of face recognition, one recognizes and evaluates a face from a general, qualitative understanding. A face is very dynamic and complex. It is almost impossible to define fixed, meaningful measurement points on it. We often hear comments such as, ''It would be better if the zygomas were a little bit higher.'' This kind of statement gives us the idea that our evaluation of a face is based on the general sense of three-dimensional form in our mind. Thus we should try to reconstruct the three-dimensional form, specifically the ones before and after the operation, in the operating surgeon's mind as well as in the patient's mind. Surgeons perform operations from their mental image of volume change to be made, not from a series of numbers or words. This is precisely the reason that pictures is much better than words in describing operative procedures. Even in the evaluation of an operative result, it is easier to identify the results by comparing the preoperative and the postoperative photos. A Chinese proverb says, ''A picture is worth a thousand words.'' Due to the development of computer graphics, there are many software packages available in three-dimensional graphic reconstruction of craniofacial surgery. Even though a gap exists between the picture produced by a computer and the result a plastic surgeon can achieve, a three-dimensional graph is very useful for plastic surgeons in the design, performance, and evaluation of the operation. However, the pictures produced by a computer are sometimes so pretty that they may mislead the patient to an unrealistic expectation.

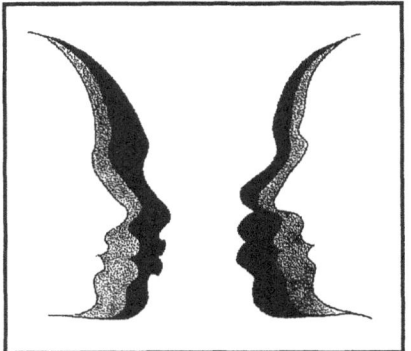

Patient Selection

Aesthetic craniofacial surgery is relatively complex and skill intensive, so patient selection is very important. Several areas should be considered in patient selection:

Psychological Factors

There is no patient whose sole purpose for the operation is aesthetics. There are always other motivations and intentions. Some want to be more attractive to elevate their position among their peers. Others attribute difficulties in their marriage or career to their appearance. In addition, the requirements for and expectations about aesthetic craniofacial surgery are different among individual patients. Therefore, plastic surgeons need to have an in-depth understanding of the patient's psychological situation before the operation.

Different patients have different concepts about beauty. Most probably, the patient's concept of beauty is not the same as that of the doctor. The plastic surgeon should discuss the expectations of the patient and offer some suggestions. The surgeon should never try to persuade the patient to accept a certain aesthetic judgment.

Computer-generated, three-dimensional graphs are used mainly in operative design by the plastic surgeon and in understanding of the procedures and results by the patient. The surgeon should emphasize that the graph produced by computer is a simulated result of the operation. It is not a real operative result simply because a cranium-face is a complex structure influenced by many factors.

Physical Factors

First, the surgeon should determine if the patient's health can withstand the kind of the aesthetic operation he or she desires. Attention should be paid to the patient's cardiovascular, hepatic, and renal functions. Existing dysfunction such as diabetes, immune diseases, or blood coagulating problems should be noted. Preferably, the age of the patient should be 20 or older. At that age, the patient can make the decision by himself or herself and craniofacial skeleton growth has completed.

Secondly, the surgeon should consider the feasibility of the operation. The surgeon should analyze the patient's face form, understand the major problem and seriousness of the abnormality, and formulate a preliminary scheme for the operation, balancing the operative result with the risk involved.

Other considerations include ethical effect, the attitudes of the patient's relatives, and the cost of the operation.

Generally, an ideal aesthetic craniofacial surgery patient should be mentally and emotionally stable and have an optimistic attitude toward life. The primary motivation for the operation is for aesthetics, and their expectation of the operation is clear and realistic. The patient should not have serious diseases or conditions that can cause possible complications. The operation should have a large chance of success. The result of the operation is ethically acceptable. The patient's relatives, such as husband or wife, should be informed of the operation. The patient should have the ability to bear the cost of the operation.

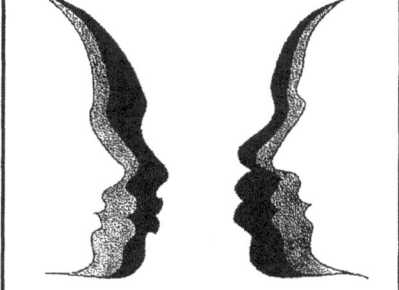

5

Surgical Preparation

The prerequisite for the success of any surgical treatment is proper presurgery preparation. The preparation involves patients and their relatives, as well as surgeons and nurses.

Preparation of Patients and Relatives

1. Familiarize the patient with the hospital environment and relieve their anxiety.
2. Take photographs of the patient's head and face in a few standard poses. Take specific photos that demonstrate the defects clearly. Record parameters, such as light, aperture, speed, distance, and film used in the photo-taking process.
3. Take an x-ray and perform computerized tomography (CT) or magnetic resonance imaging (MRI) examination of the craniofacial skeleton. If possible, reconstruct a three-dimensional image of the patient's head from the CT or MRI data.
4. Perform an overall physical examination and biochemical tests. Any unfavorable circumstances to the operation should be corrected.
5. Obtain a blood test and cross-matching.
6. Explain to the patient the operation procedures, possible complications during and after the operation, and the corresponding measures. Solicit their cooperation in the operation.
7. Get the preoperative signature from the patient.
8. Preparation of the incisions for different areas on the head and face:
   a. Bicoronal and hairline incisions—Two days before the operation, the male patient will have his head shaved. For the female patient, a 1 cm area should be shaved along the

planned incision and the head washed twice that day. The next day, her hair should be plaited along the incision and her head soaked with ethyl alcohol three times for 20 minutes each. After the last soak, wrap the head with a sterile wrapper. The reason for shaving the head two days before the operation is to have the hair grow back a little bit. The short stab will define clearly the direction of hair growth and prevent the operative incision from damaging hair papillae and leaving a bald line.

b. Incisions near eyes—Use antibiotic ointment on the eyes several times a day and do not apply makeup to the face two days before the operation.

c. Incisions in nostrils—Cut vibrissa and use antibiotic liquid in nasal cavity several times a day for two days before the operation. Any nasosinusitis should be corrected.

d. Intraoral incisions—Brush teeth after each meal for two days prior to the operation and rinse the mouth with Dobell's solution several times a day. Any decayed teeth and gingivitis should be treated.

e. Facial skin incisions—Cleanse the face using neutral soap several times a day. Do not use makeup during the two days before the operation. Any skin furuncles or infections should be treated.

9. Begin to administer antibiotic orally or intravenously the day before the operation.

Preparation of Doctors and Nurses

1. Doctors and nurses should establish a good relationship with the patient during the preoperative preparations. Gaining the full trust of the patient is an essential element for a successful operation.

2. Further understand the patient's psychological situation. Find out any existing mental problems.

3. Carefully study the patient's face. In collaboration with the anesthetist and nurses, formulate a detailed operative plan.

a. Anesthetic methods—Anesthesia in aesthetic craniofacial surgery is mainly intratracheal anesthesia through the nostril or the mouth. Since the plastic surgeons are operating in close proximity to the tube, the patient's head is moved frequently and the tracheal tube may slip out, the fixation of tracheal tube is very important. Normally, endotracheal intubation can be done through either the oral or the nasal route. For oral intubation, endotracheal tube is either wired to the maxillary teeth or the mandibular teeth (Fig. 5-1(a)). Nasotracheal intubation is generally used for the operation that involves occlusal correction. The nasotracheal tube is fixed by suturing it to the nasal septum and the forehead scalp (Fig. 5-1(b)).

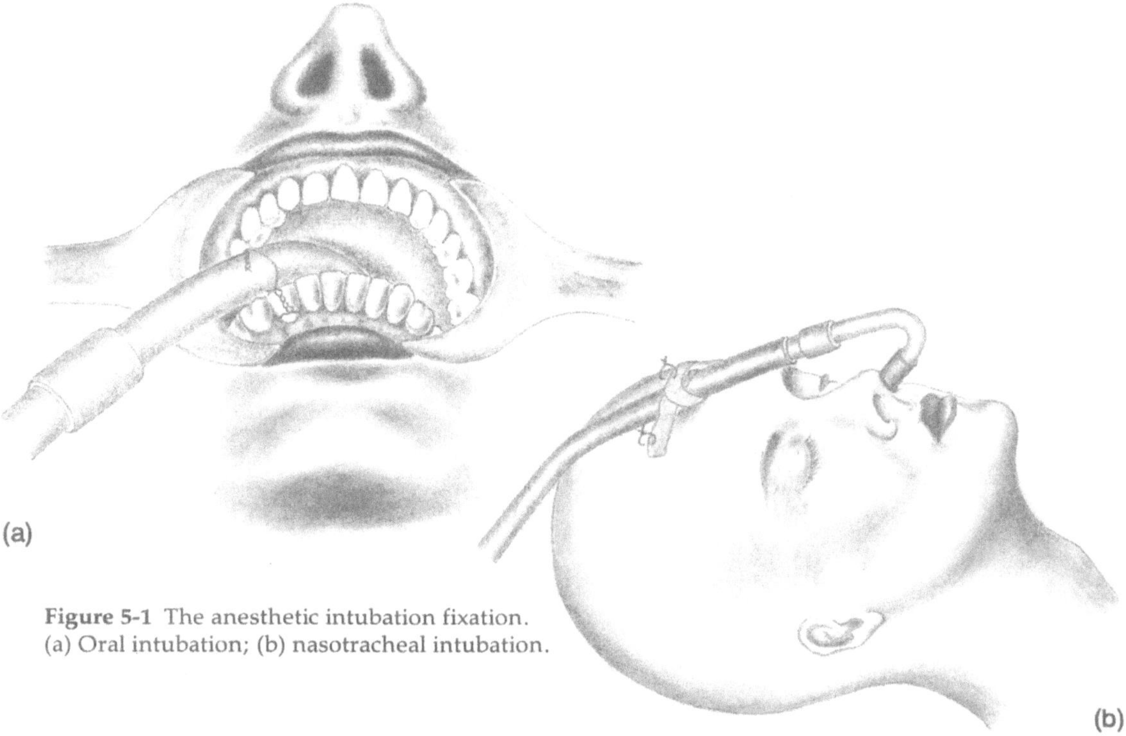

(a)

Figure 5-1 The anesthetic intubation fixation.
(a) Oral intubation; (b) nasotracheal intubation.

(b)

b. Patient's position—The patient should be placed in a com-
fortable position with the head higher than the legs. The
neck extends back slightly, the hips and the knees are
slightly flexed. This position reduces the blood pressure
in the head and reduces blood loss during the operation
(Fig. 5-2).

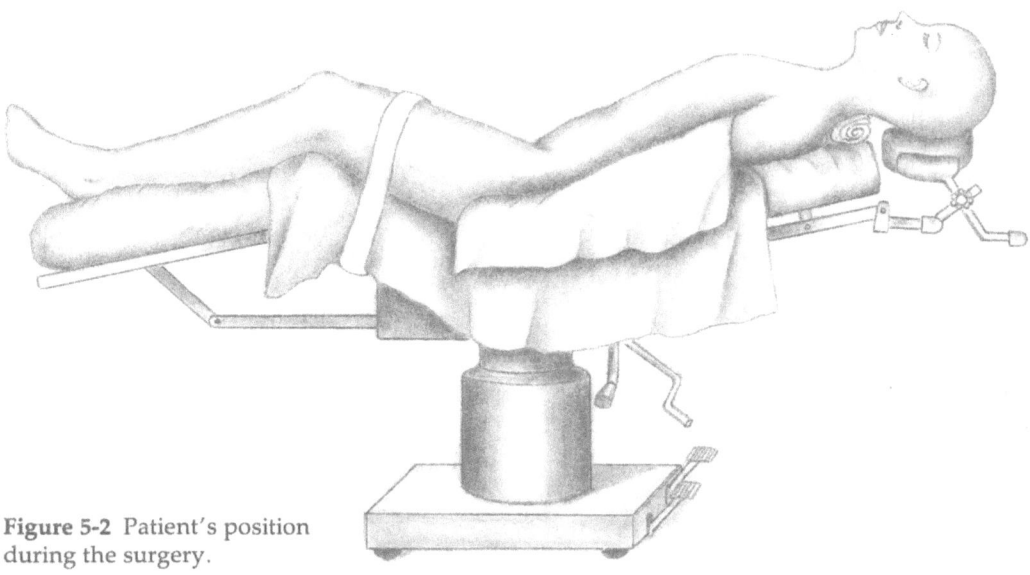

Figure 5-2 Patient's position
during the surgery.

c. Position of the surgical team—The anesthetist and operative surgeons may interfere with each other, as both anesthesia and surgery are performed in the limited space on the patient's head. The position of each medical team member should be determined by factors such as the area of operation on the patient, the anesthesia method used, and the handedness of the operative surgeon (Figs. 5-3, 5-4, 5-5).

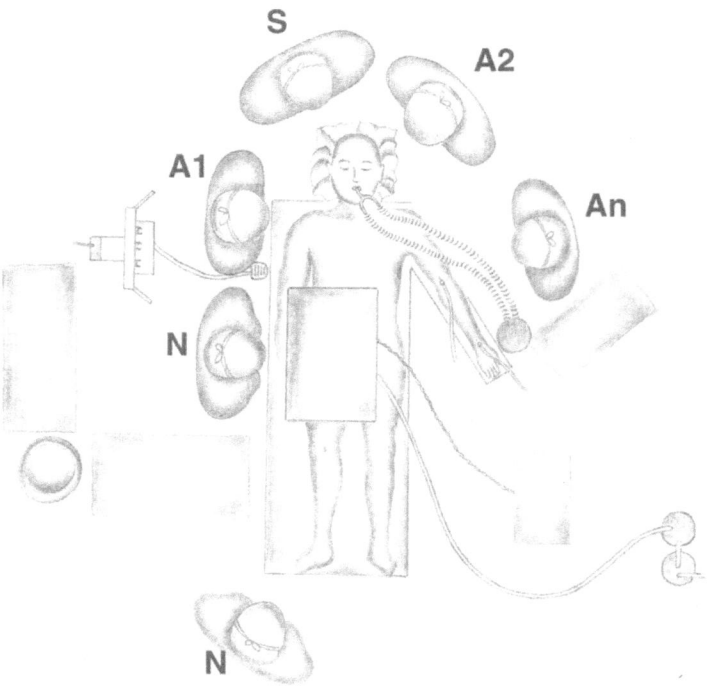

Figure 5-3 The positioning of the anesthesia-surgical team for craniofacial procedures. An: Anesthesiologist; S: surgeon; A1: first assistant; A2: second assistant; N: nurse.

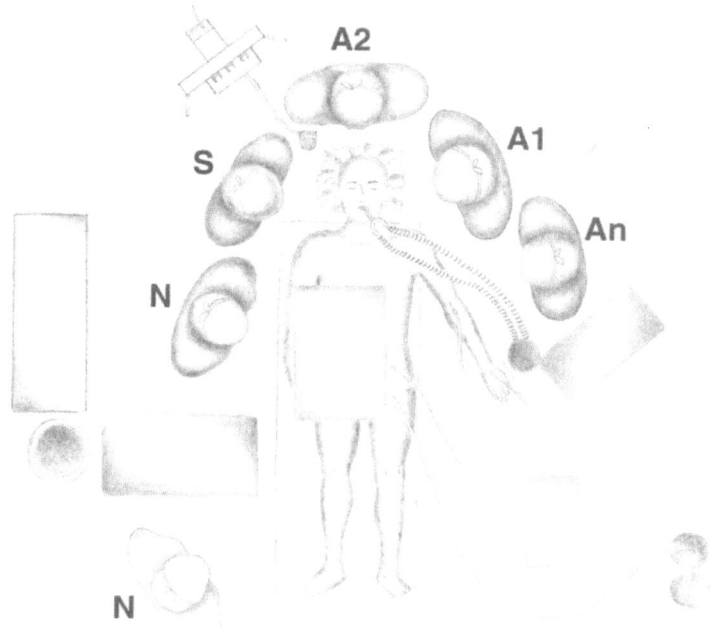

Figure 5-4 The positioning of the anesthesia-surgical team for maxillofacial procedures. An: Anesthesiologist; S: surgeon; A1: first assistant; A2: second assistant; N: nurse.

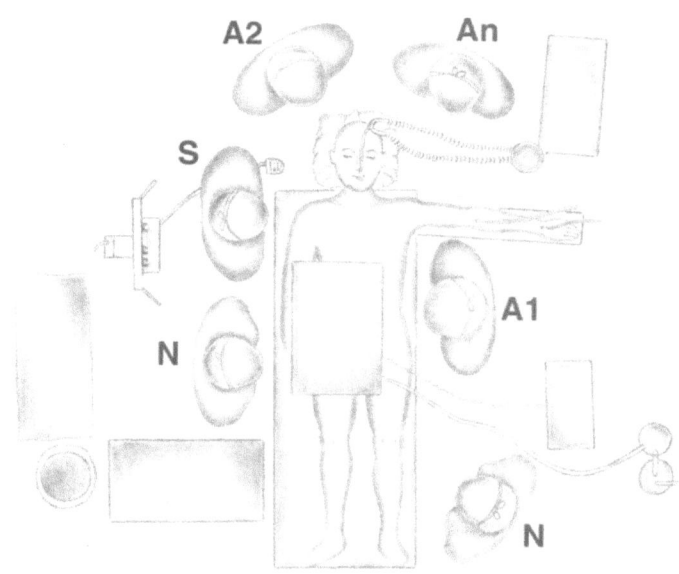

Figure 5-5 The positioning of anesthesia-surgical team for mandibular procedures. An: Anesthesiologist; S: surgeon; A1: first assistant; A2: second assistant; N: nurse.

d. Define approaches and donor of bone—The approach chosen should benefit the osteotomies and avoid obvious scars (Fig. 5-6). There are different implant materials for aesthetic craniofacial surgery, such as autograft, allotransplant, and synthetic materials. Some problems exist with the use of allotransplant and synthetic materials: they tend to have large absorption and hard mergence into the receptors. They may even be rejected psychologically by some patients. Autograft, without those problems, is still the preferred material in aesthetic craniofacial surgery. The position and size of donor bone should be determined before the operation (Figs. 5-7, 5-8, 5-9, 5-10).

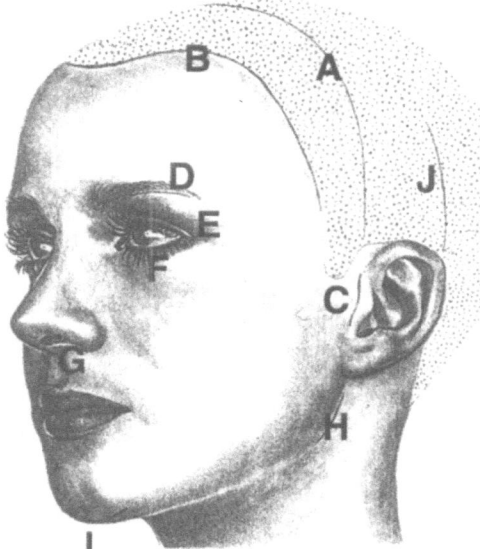

(A) Coronal scalp incision
(B) frontal hairline incision
(C) preauricular incision
(D) infrabrow incision
(E) upper blepharoplasty incision
(G) labio-alar groove incision
(H) posterior mandibular angle incision
(I) submental incision
(J) cranial bone harvesting incision

(K) Upper buccal sulcus incision
(L) lower buccal sulcus incision
(M) posterior buccal fat pad mucosal incision
(N) intranasal intercartilaginous incision
(O) intranasal infracartilaginous incision
(P) alar rim incision
(Q) transmembranous columella incision
(R) transcolumella incision
(S) palatal mucosal incision

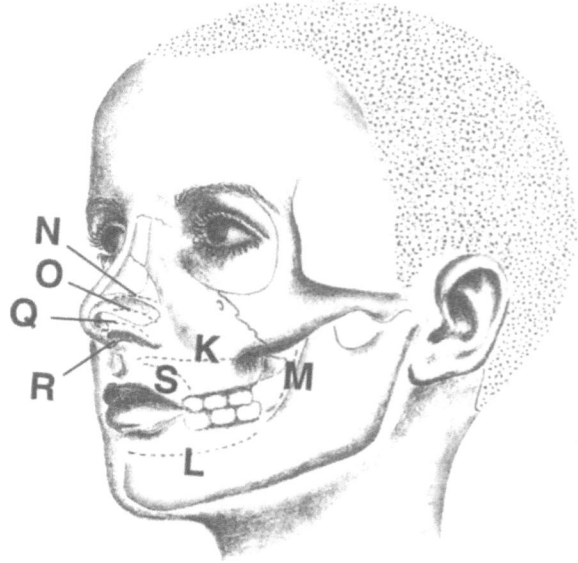

Figure 5-6 Surgical approaches of craniofacial surgery (a) and (b).

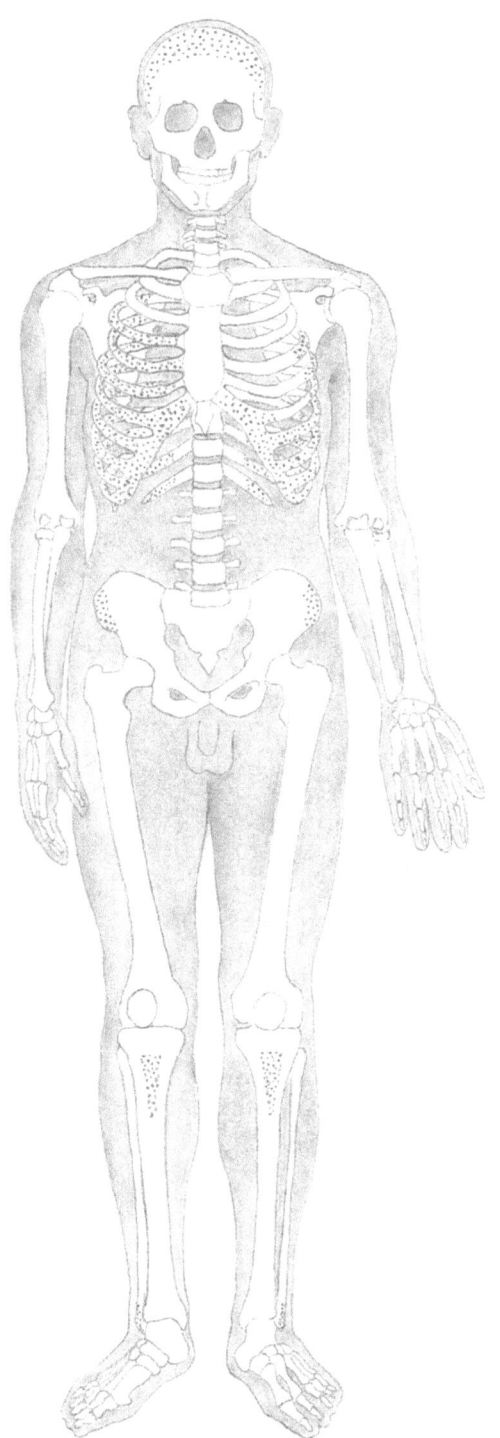

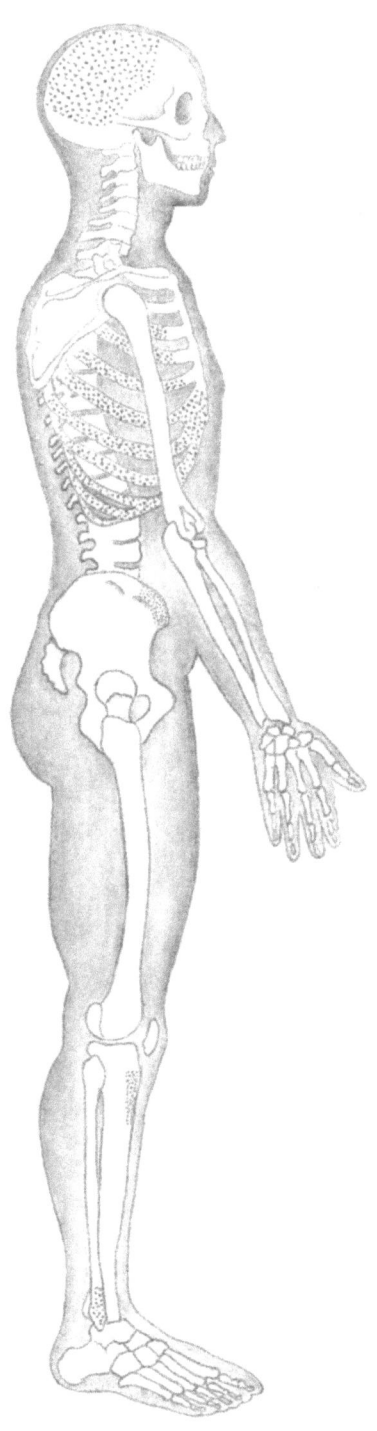

Figure 5-7 The stippled areas illustrate the osseous donor sites on frontal view.

Figure 5-8 The stippled areas illustrate the osseous donor sites on lateral view.

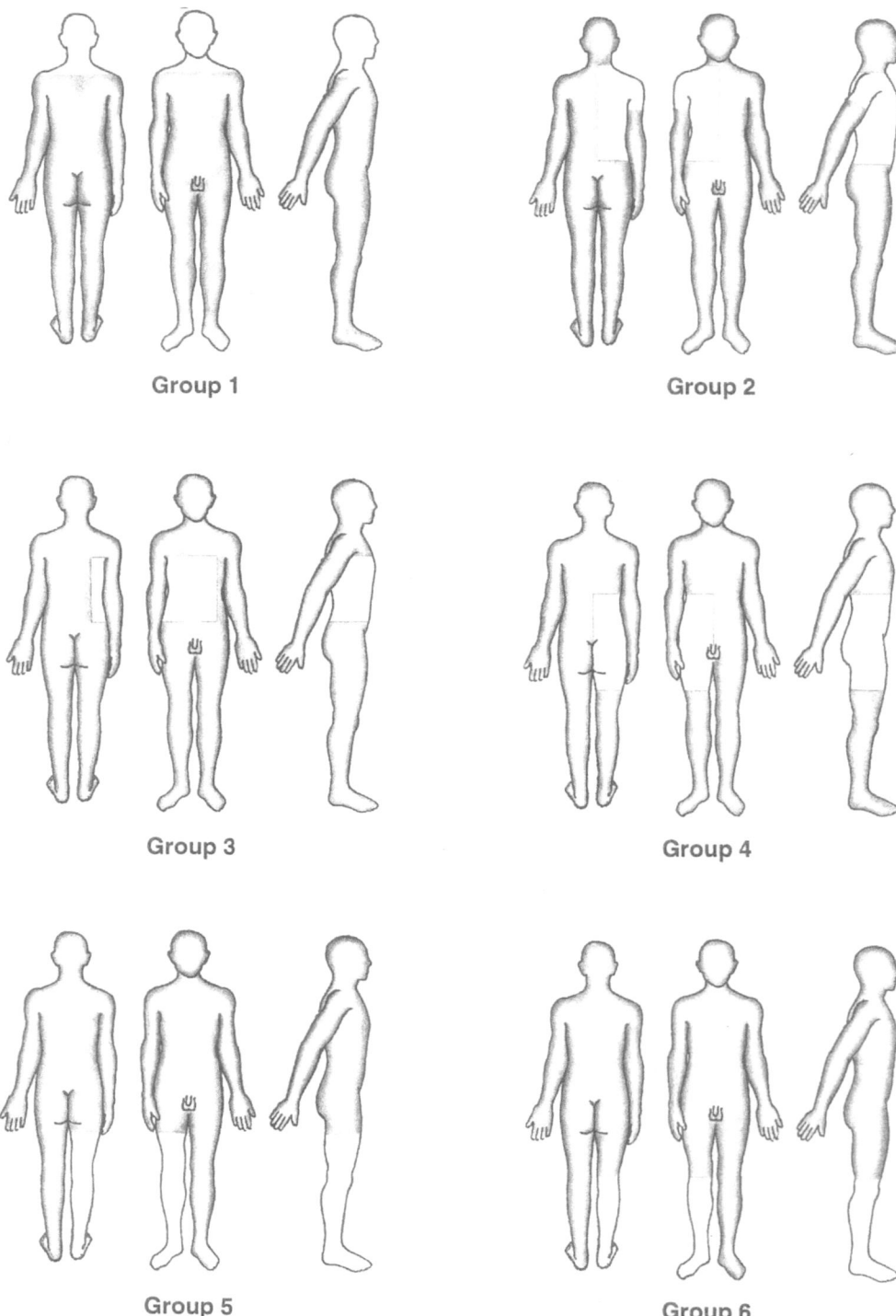

Figure 5-9 The sterile fields of craniofacial surgery and bone harvest. Group 1: sterile field of craniofacial surgery. Group 2: sterile field of the lateral rib harvest. Group 3: sterile field of the frontal rib harvest. Group 4: sterile field of the iliac bone harvest. Group 5: sterile field of the tibial bone harvest. Group 6: sterile field of the lateral malleolar bone harvest.

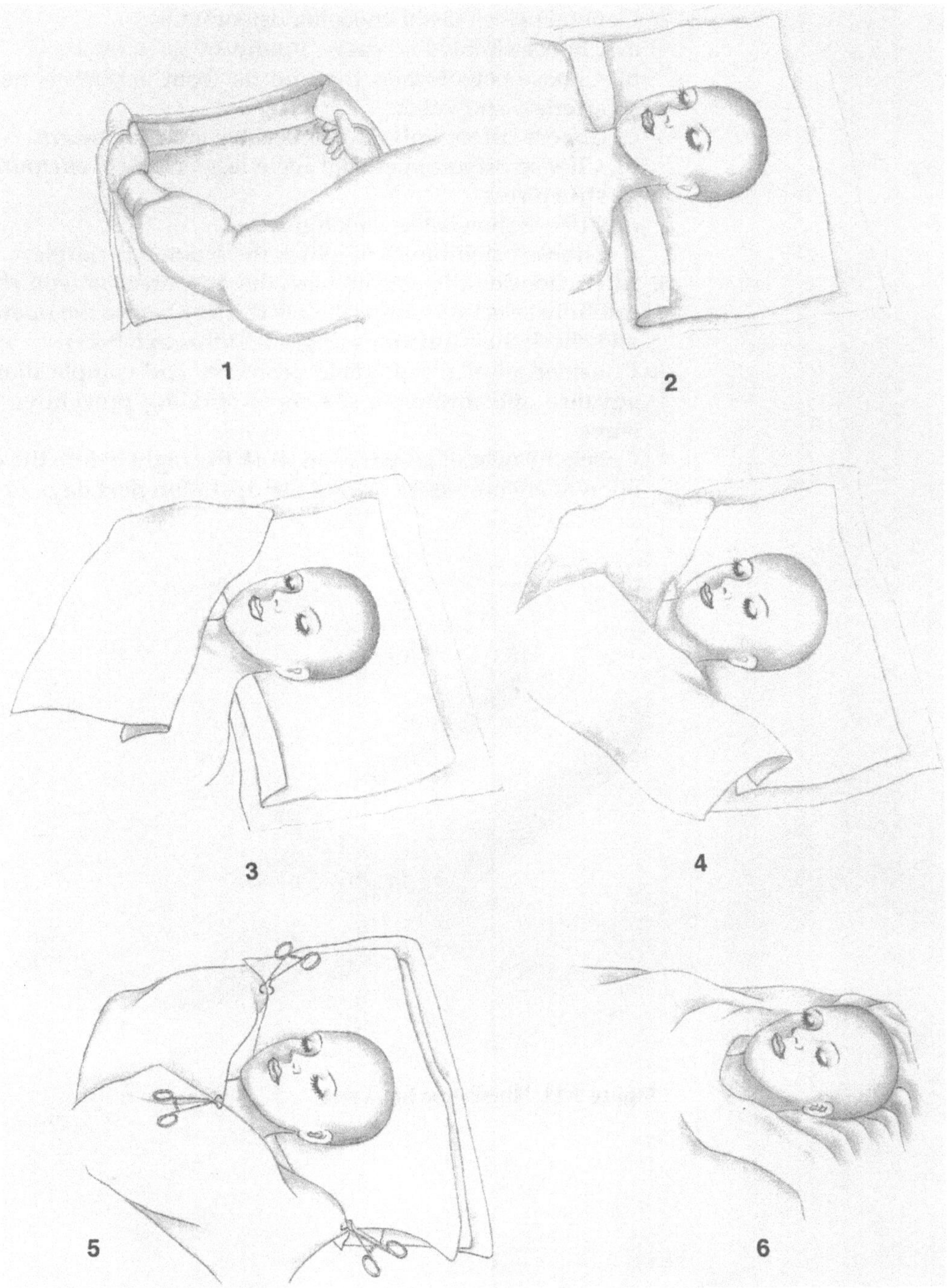

Figure 5-10 The draping technique for craniofacial surgery.

4. General principles of choosing osteotomies:
   a. Choose simple and easy-to-perform osteotomies.
   b. Choose osteotomies that are far from important nerves, arteries, and veins.
   c. Choose osteotomies that are stable after relocation.
   d. Choose osteotomies that have less effect on surrounding structures.
   e. Choose the visible osteotomies.
   f. Choose osteotomies in which the fixation is simple.
5. After choosing the osteotomies, the operative surgeon should carefully select the surgical tools the day before the operation and check their functions (Figs. 5-11 through 5-25).
6. Consider all of the possible problems and complications in advance and formulate the corresponding preventive measures.
7. Check the overall preparation work the night before the operation to ensure safety during the operation next day.

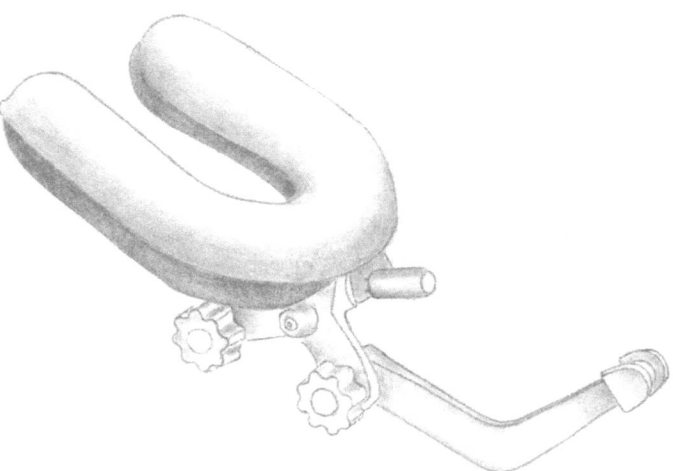

Figure 5-11 Horseshoe head rest.

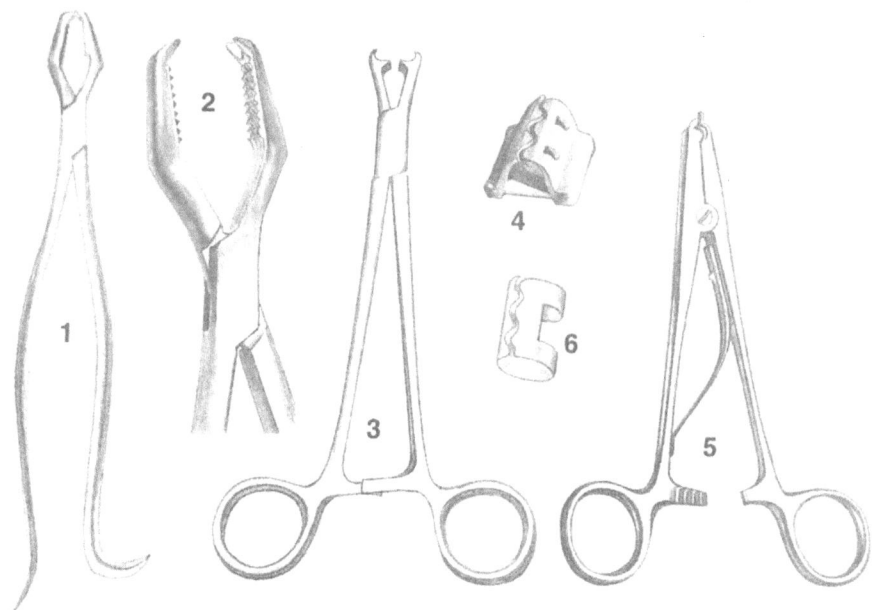

Figure 5-12 (1) Lane bone-holding forceps; (2) Lane bone-holding forceps tip; (3) LeRoy scalp clip applying forceps; (4) LeRoy disposable scalp clip; (5) Raney scalp clip applying forceps; (6) Raney stainless steel scalp clip.

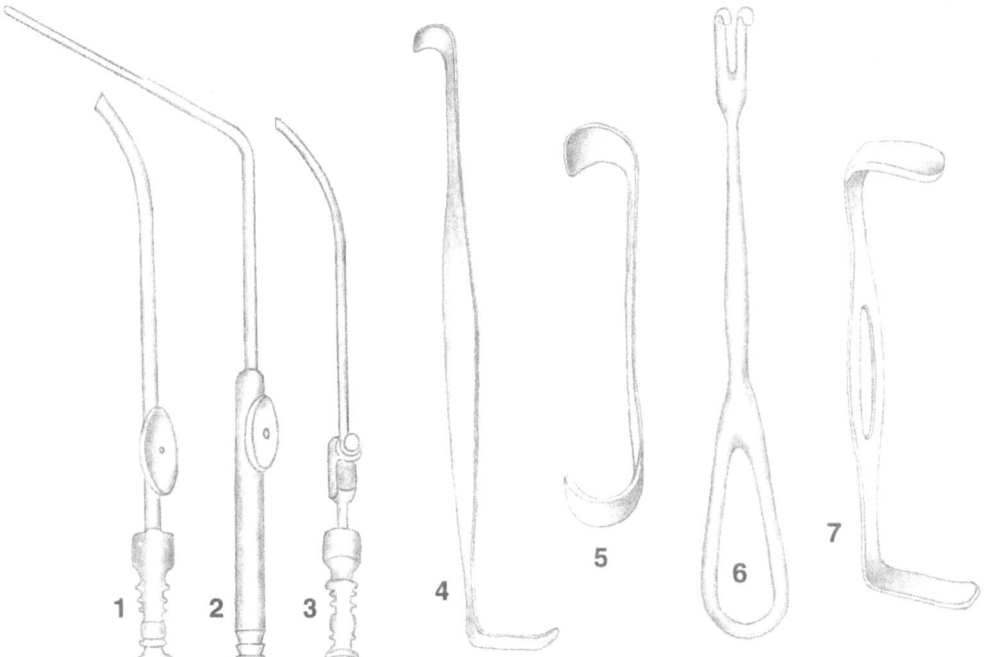

Figure 5-13 (1) Adson suction tube; (2) Sachs suction tube; (3) Frazier suction tube; (4) Senn retractor; (5) Parker retractor; (6) small rake retractor; (7) U.S. retractor.

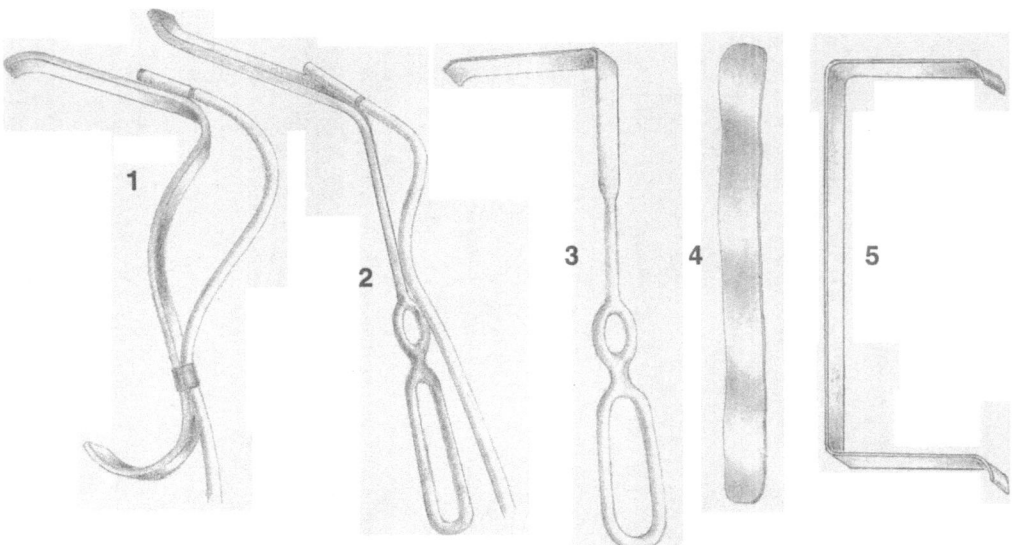

Figure 5-14 (1) Lighted lateral ramus retractor; (2) lighted medial ramus retractor; (3) retractor; (4) malleable retractor; (5) retractor.

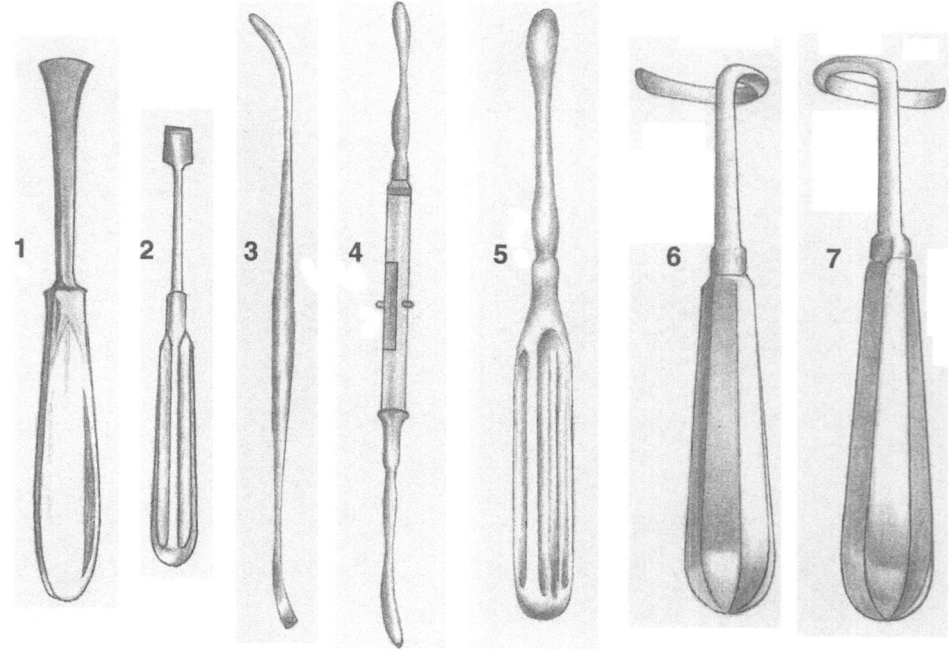

Figure 5-15 (1) Cushing elevator, wide square edge; (2) Adson elevator, chisel edge; (3) Penfield elevator; (4) staphylorraphy elevator; (5) Adson elevator, curved blunt edge; (6) left Doyen rib raspatory; (7) right Doyen rib raspatory.

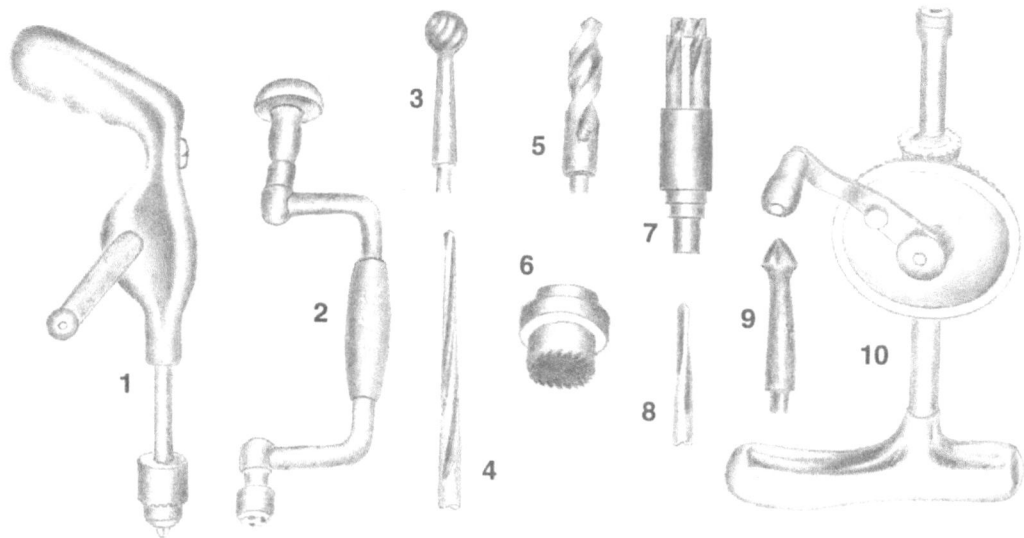

Figure 5-16 (1) Zimmer hand drill; (2) Hudson brace; (3) Mckenzie enlarging burr; (4) Long steel drill; (5) Mckenzie perforator drill; (6) skull trephine; (7) skull perforator; (8) short steel drill; (9) Adson perforating burr; (10) Stille cranial drill.

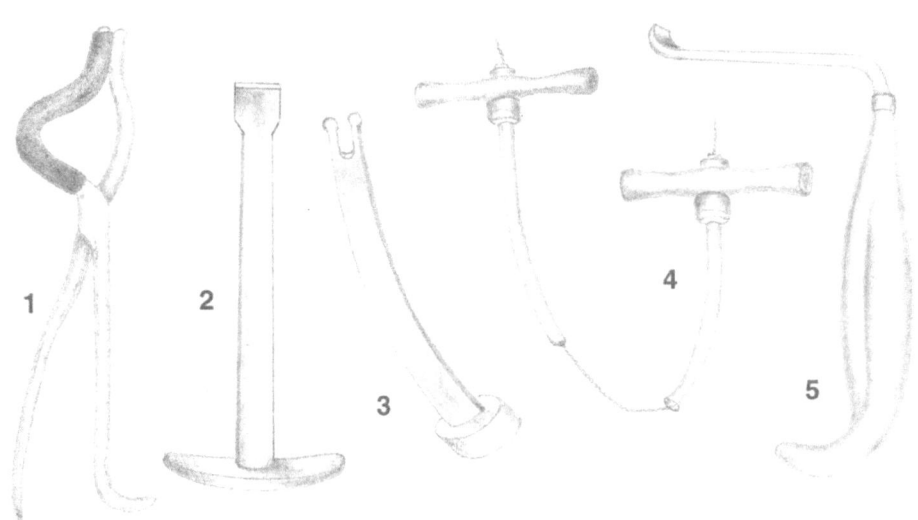

Figure 5-17 (1) Rowe disimpaction forceps with rubber protector; (2) Dautrey osteotome; (3) curved double-ball osteotome; (4) Gigli saw and handle with malleable guard; (5) bone elevator.

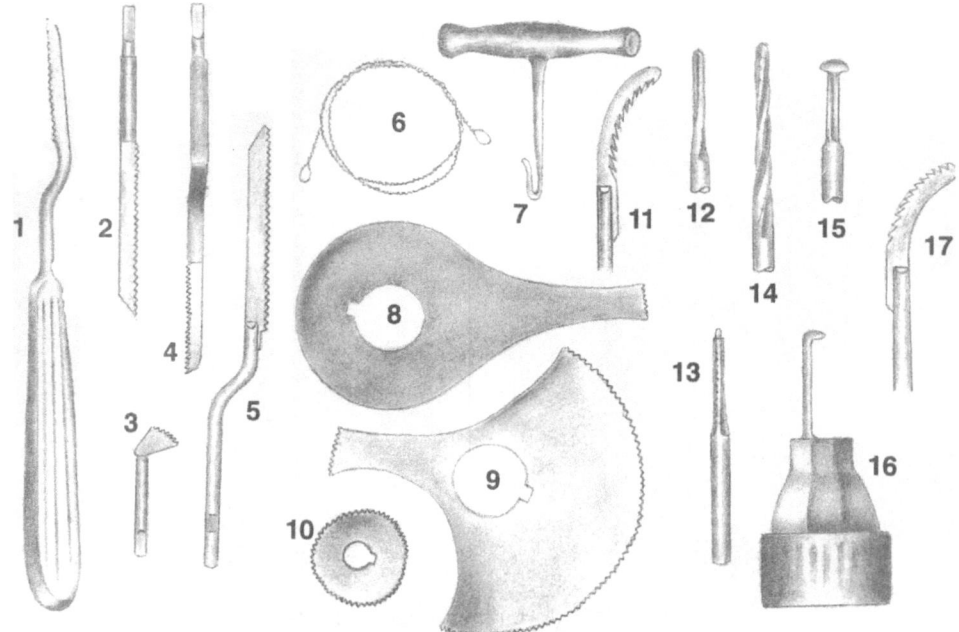

Figure 5-18 (1) Joseph saw; (2) regular saw blade; (3) right-angle oscillating saw blade; (4) right offset saw blade; (5) down offset saw blade; (6) Gigli saw blade; (7) Gigli saw handle; (8) oscillating saw blade, deep narrow blade; (9) oscillating saw blade, large blade; (1) rotary saw blade; (11) reciprocating saw blade, curved blade; (12) short saw-like steel burr; (13) neuro blade; (14) long steel burr; (15) neuro blade with guard; (16) dura guard; (17) reciprocating saw blade, curved blade.

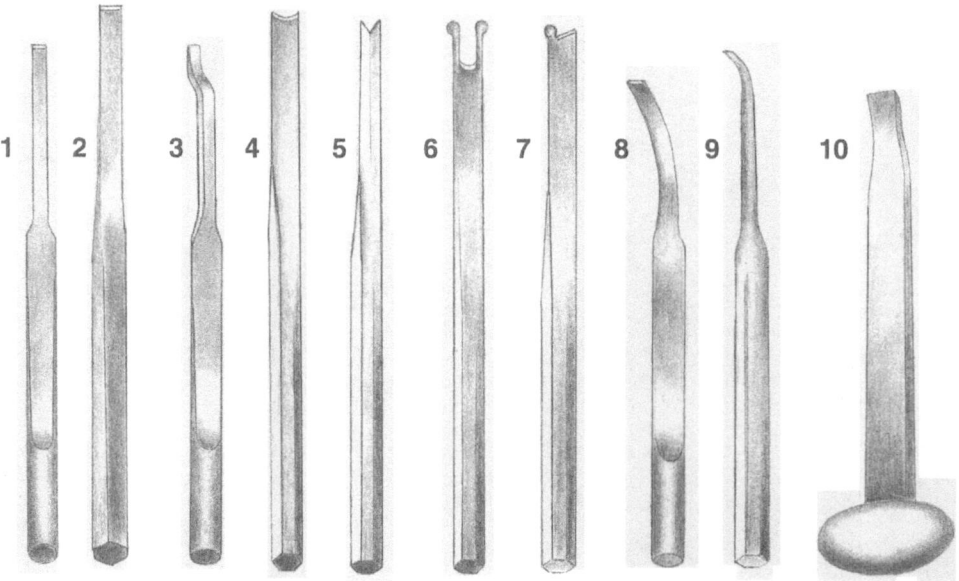

Figure 5-19 (1) Sheehan nasal chisel; (2) Cottle chisel; (3) down offset osteotome; (4) straight osteotome, curved edge; (5) straight osteotome, angular edge; (6) double-ball osteotome; (7) single-ball osteotome; (8) curved osteotome; (9) curved osteotome; (10) Kawamoto osteotome.

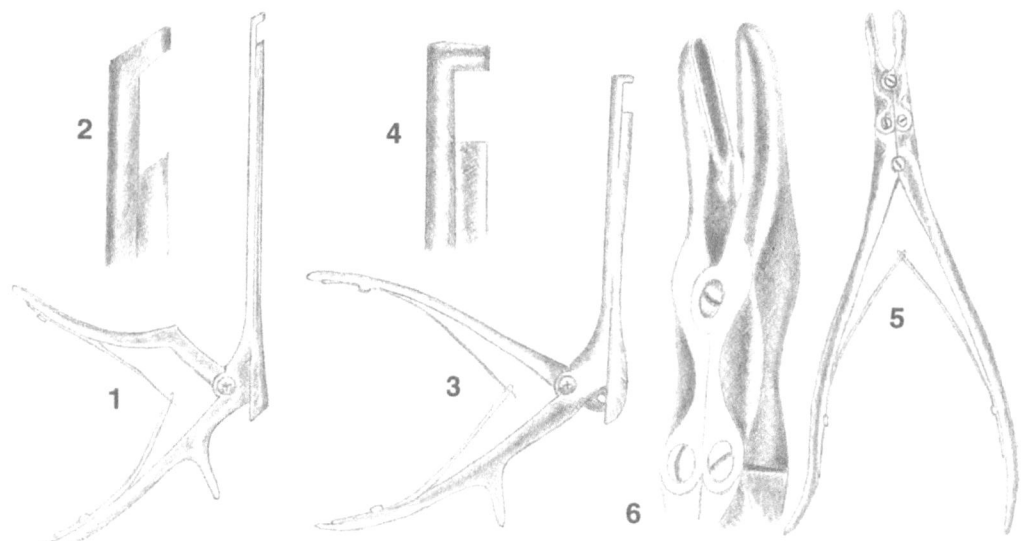

Figure 5-20 (1) Spurling Kerrison rongeur 40 degree forward-angle jaw; (2) Spurling Kerrison rongeur tip; (3) Whitcomb Kerrison laminectomy rongeur; (4) Whitcomb Kerrison laminectomy rongeur tip; (5) Smith-Petersen laminectomy rongeur; (6) Smith-Petersen laminectomy rongeur tip.

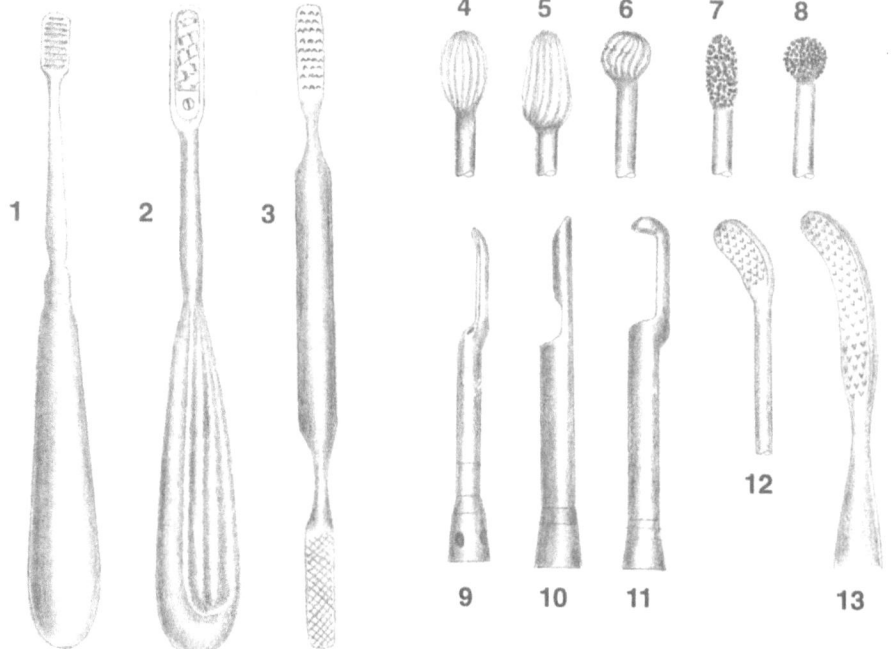

Figure 5-21 (1) Lewis rasp; (2) Rubin planer with replaceable blade; (3) Fomon rasp; (4) oval burr; (5) burr; (b) ball burr; (7) diamond burr, oval; (8) diamond burr, ball; (9) rhinoplasty guard; (10) tissue protector guard; (11) laminectomy burr guard; (12) reciprocating rasp, curved; (13) Lewis rasp, curved.

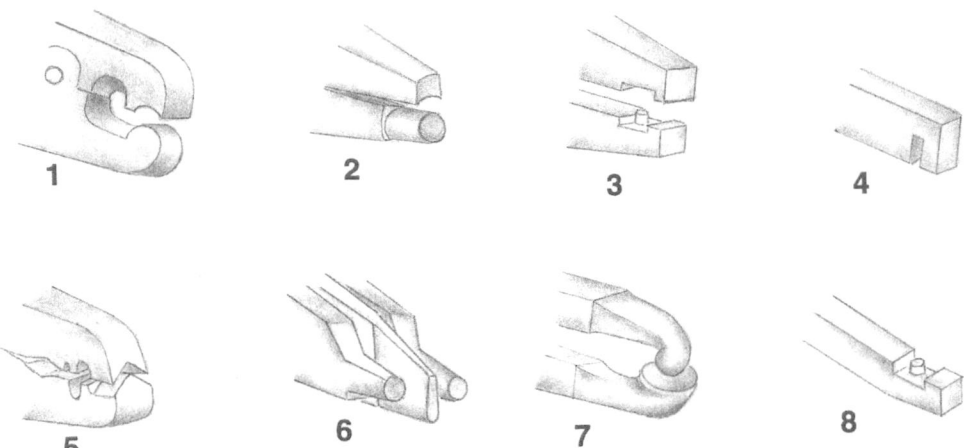

Figure 5-22 (1) Tubular bending pliers tip; (2) horizontal bending pliers tip; (3) plate-bending pliers tip; (4) plate-bending iron end; (5) right-angle bending pliers tip; (6) three-prong bending pliers tip; (7) sphere-bending pliers tip; (8) bending iron end.

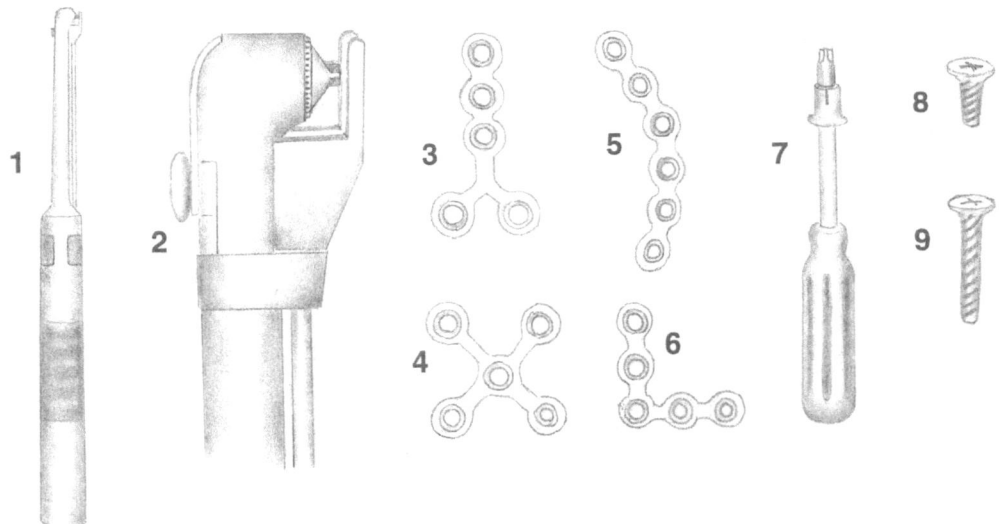

Figure 5-23 (1) Right-angle screwdriver; (2) right-angle screwdriver head; (3) Y-shaped miniplate; (4) X-shaped miniplate; (5) C-shaped miniplate; (6) L-shaped miniplate; (7) screwdriver with screw holder; (8) screw, short; (9) screw, long.

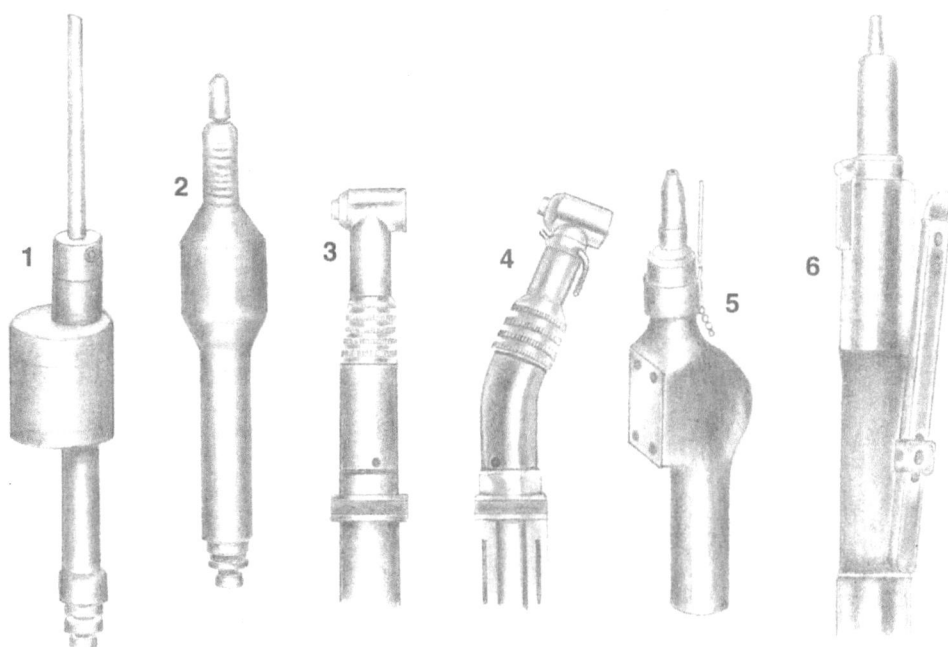

Figure 5-24 (1) Oscillating saw attachment; (2) reciprocating saw attachment; (3) air drill 100 attachment, 90° angle; (4) air drill 100 attachment, 70° angle; (5) reciprocating saw attachment with irrigation; (6) Air drill 100 attachment.

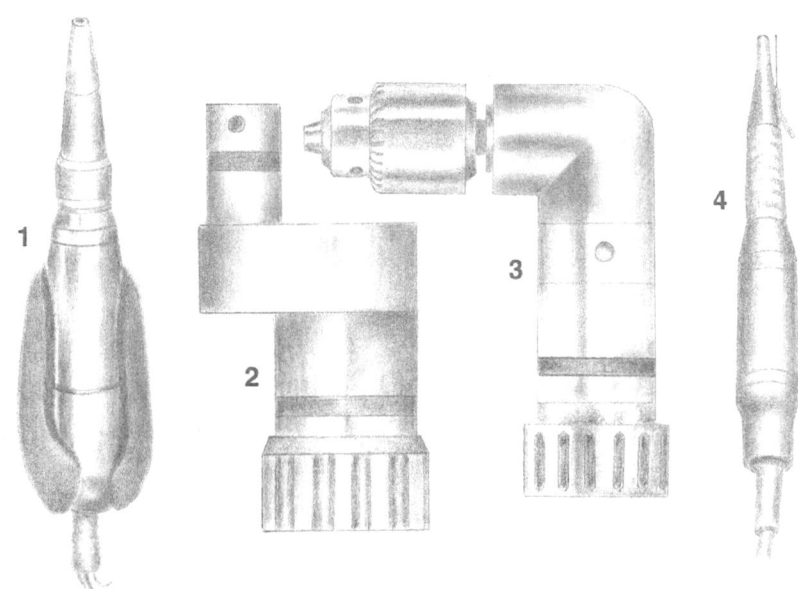

Figure 5-25 (1) Acrotorque hand engine; (2) oscillating saw attachment; (3) wire and pin driver; (4) Aesculap Microtron drill with irrigation.

6

Osteotomy
Methods

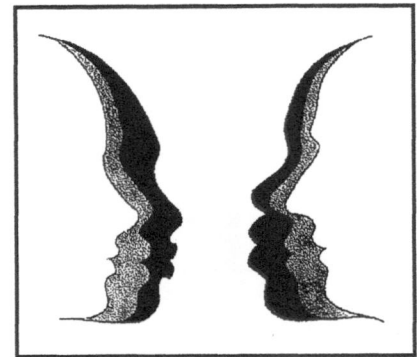

From a sculptor's point of view, each part of the skull contributes significantly to the contour of the face. For convenience in operative designs and communication with the patient, a skull is usually divided into several significant areas (Fig. 6-1).

Changing a facial form is achieved first by the osteotomy design and then the movement of the bone blocks. Since there are a large variety osteotomy methods, we are illustrating only those most frequently used.

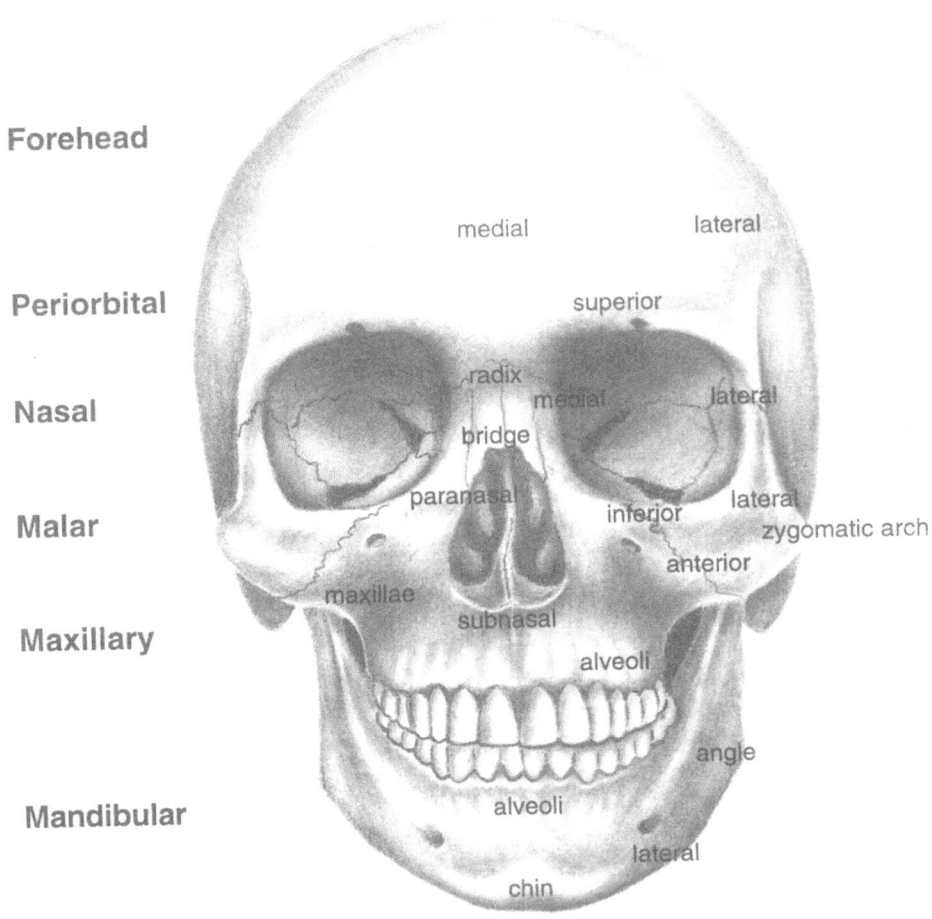

Figure 6–1 (1) Frontal head (medial, lateral); (2) periorbital (superior, lateral, inferior); (3) nasal (radix, bridge, subnasal, paranasal); (4) malar (anterior, lateral, zygomatic arch); (5) maxillary (alveoli, maxillae); (6) mandibular (chin, lateral, alveoli, angle).

Method

The scalp incision is made at the posterior parietal area. The periosteum is elevated from the cranium. An outline of a predetermined width and length of donor bone is marked. With a small rotary saw, the outline is cut down to the diploe. Then a Gigli saw is inserted into the outline and performed in seesaw fashion to harvest the bone graft (Fig. 6-2).

Method

The cranial bone is exposed via the coronal incision. The burr hole can be drilled by a Hudson's brace or a hand engine. After the outer table is penetrated, care must be taken and the progress of the drilling should be checked from time to time. When the inner table is penetrated, a slight change in the feel of the drill may be detected and the skull perforator is exchanged. The hole is enlarged until it is parallel-sided (Fig. 6-3).

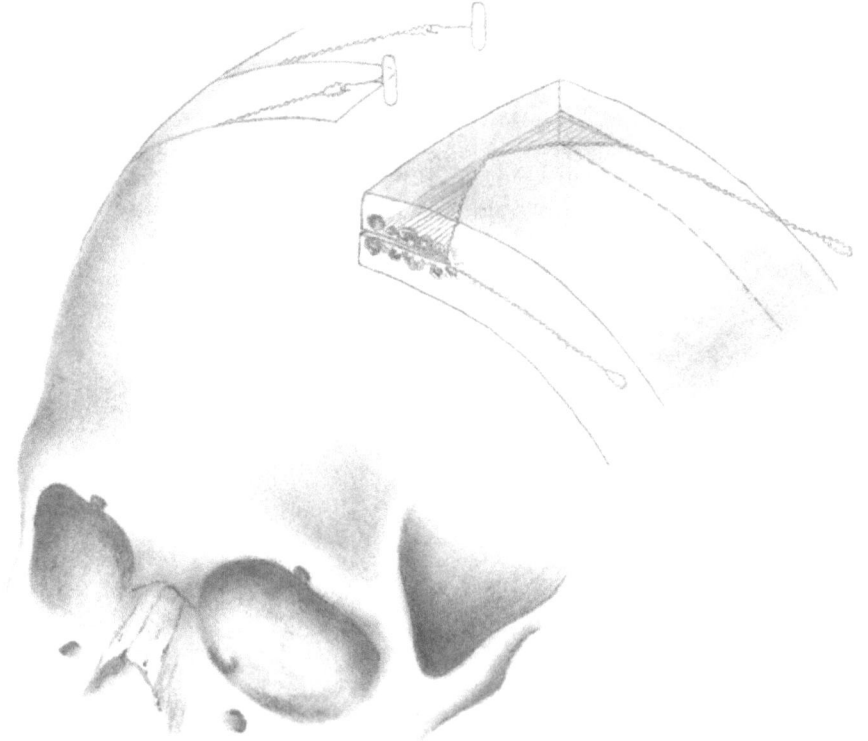

Figure 6–2

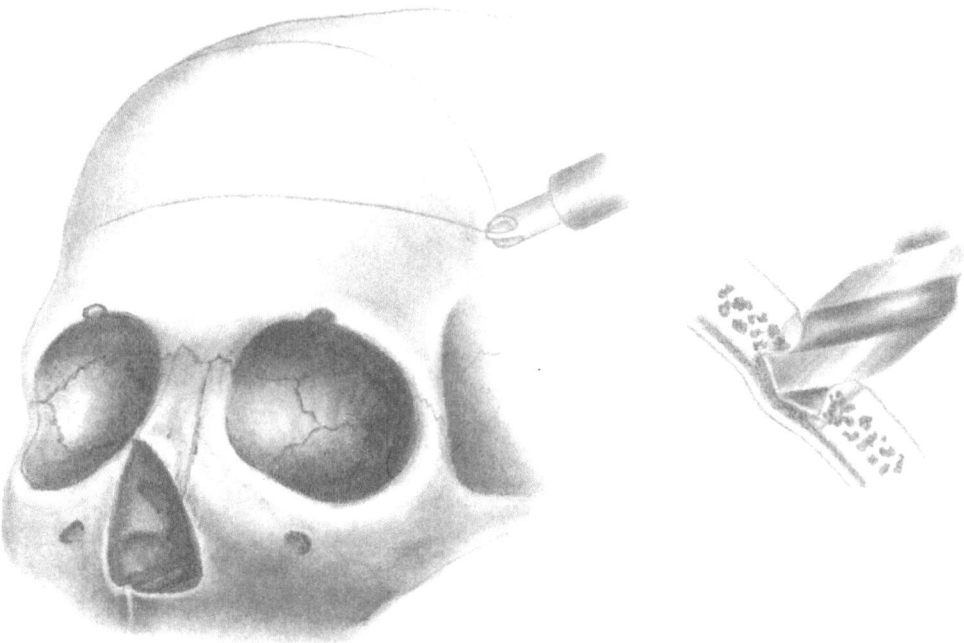

Figure 6–3

Method

The coronal incision is made and the periosteum is elevated from the frontal head. The burr holes are drilled about 6 cm apart, along the line of the craniotomy. With a blunt curved Adson periosteal elevator, the dura is gently separated from the bone between the burr holes. The craniotomy is completed using a neuro blade with a dura guard (Fig. 6-4).

Method

This osteotomy is performed horizontally at the level just above the orbital roof. During this procedure, the brain is protected by a malleable retractor (Fig. 6-5).

Method

After the frontal craniotomy is completed, the fossa crania anterior is exposed by retracting the brain posteriorly. Using an oscillating saw, the sagittal osteotomy medial to the medial orbital wall is performed at the desired position (Fig. 6-6).

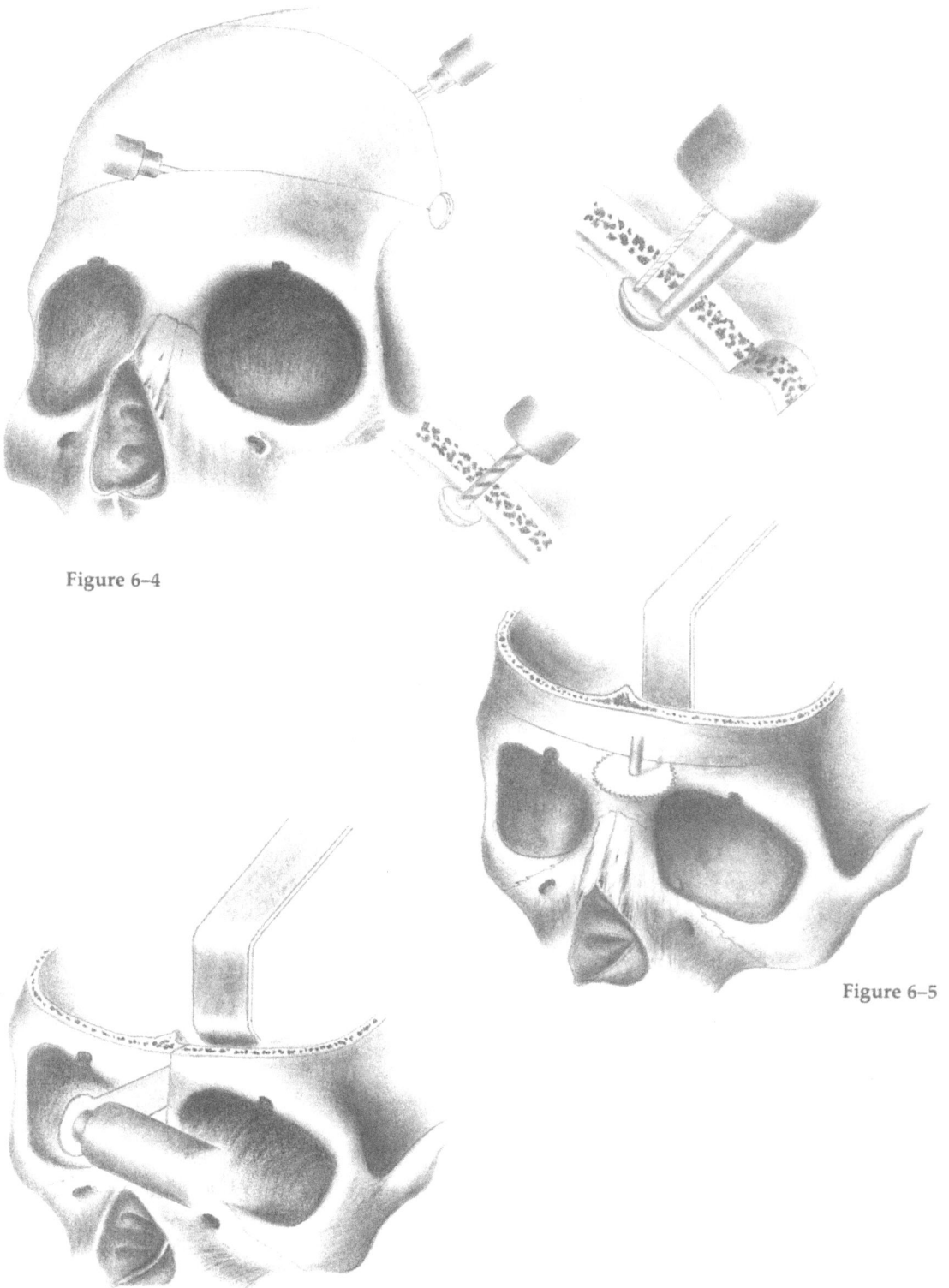

Figure 6–4

Figure 6–5

Figure 6–6

Method

A coronal incision is made. The subperiosteal dissection is extended to the level of the medial and lateral canthal ligaments. The frontal craniectomy is performed initially. After the frontal bone has been removed, the osteotomy on the orbital roof is made by a burr or an oscillating saw with intracranial and orbital protection (Fig. 6-7).

Method

After the frontal craniotomy is completed, the orbital roofs are exposed by the retraction of the brain. With the malleable retractors the brain and the orbital contents are protected. Using a reciprocating saw the osteotomy anterior to the fossa crania media is performed via the temporal fossa (Fig. 6-8).

Method

The frontal hairline incision is made in the midline. The subperiosteal dissection is done on the frontal sinus surface. An oval burr with a tissue retractor guard is inserted to perform the bone reduction. The tissue retractor guard will retract and protect the surrounding soft tissue. A common complication resulting from this procedure is the damage of the supraorbital nerve (Fig. 6-9).

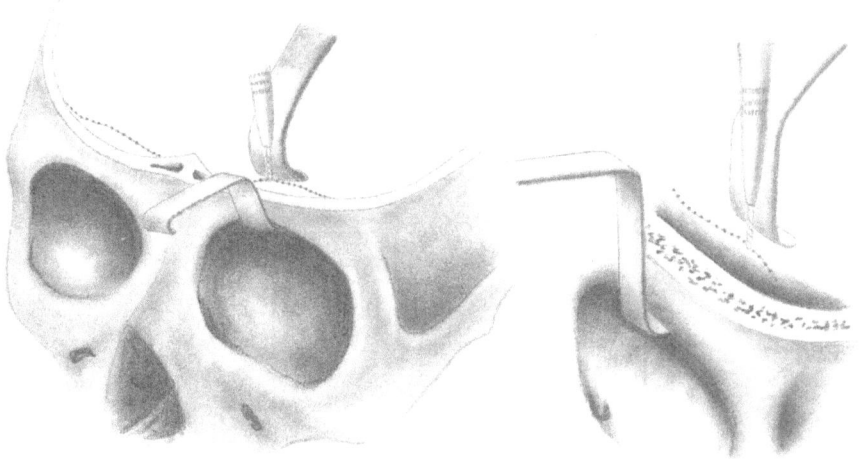

Figure 6–7

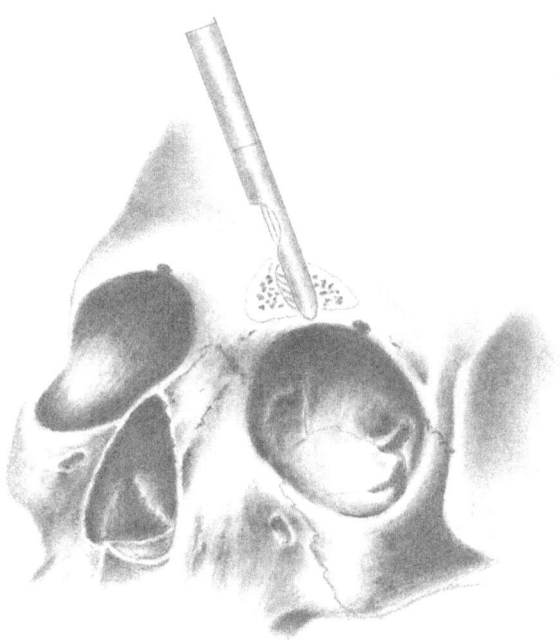

Figure 6–8

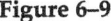

Figure 6–9

Method

A coronal incision is made and the subperiosteal dissection is continued to the medial orbital wall. With the orbital contents protected, a fine curved osteotome is inserted to cut the posterior-medial orbital wall vertically. The upper edge of the osteotome should never be placed above the level of the cribriform plate to prevent entering the anterior cranial fossa (Fig. 6-10).

Method

A nasal vestibule incision is made. With an Adson elevator, the nasal mucosa is elevated from the medial maxillary wall. Then a fine curved osteotome is used to cut the medial maxillary wall vertically posterior to the nasolacrimal tube (Fig. 6-11).

Method

The coronal incision is used to expose the medial orbital wall and the orbital floor. Then, a nasal vestibule incision provides access to the medial maxillary wall. The orbital contents are protected by a malleable retractor. A narrow curved osteotome is used to make the osteotomy behind the nasolacrimal tube, entering the orbit (Fig. 6-12).

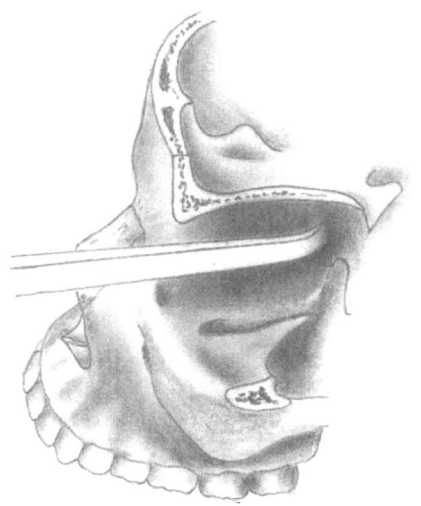

Figure 6–10

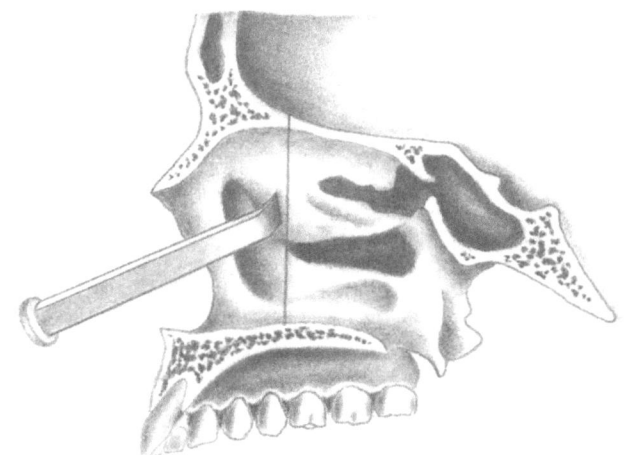

Figure 6–11

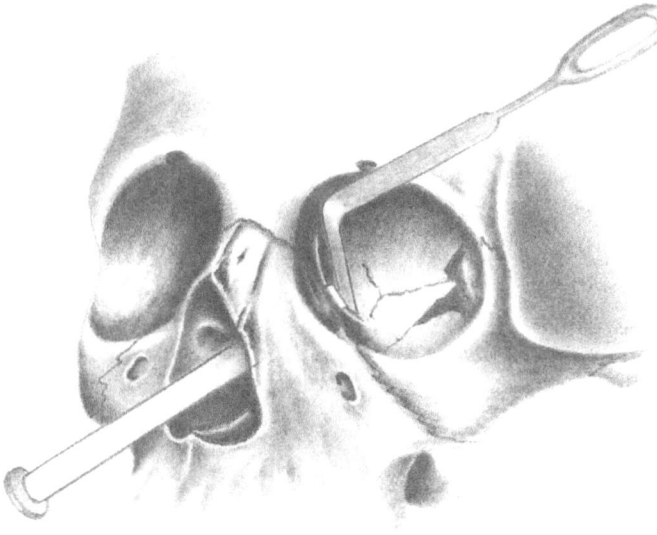

Figure 6–12

Method

The coronal incision is made for the exposure. The subperiosteal dissection is continued to the malar eminence and the temporal fossa. A hole is drilled through the lateral inferior orbital rim, entering the temporal fossa. A Gigli saw is introduced through the hole and the osteotomy in a cephalad direction is performed in a seesaw manner. By changing the pulling direction during the cutting stroke, the lateral orbital rim can be split into different forms (Fig. 6-13).

Method

The coronal incision is usually used for the access to the orbits and the zygomatic arches. Subperiosteal dissection is continued to the medial orbital wall and the zygomatic arch. With a malleable retractor, the orbital contents are protected. Using a reciprocating saw with a narrow blade, the osteotomy is directed to the inferior orbital fissure and made at the medial orbital wall. With a malleable Gigli saw guard, the Gigli saw is introduced around the zygomatic arch and the osteotomy is made at the desired position (Fig. 6-14).

Method

Exposure is obtained via a coronal incision and subperiosteal dissection is continued to the infraorbital rims. With protection of the orbital contents, a saw-like burr is used to cut the lateral portion of the orbital floor. The burr should be moved slowly in a seesaw manner and irrigation should be employed during the procedure (Fig. 6-15).

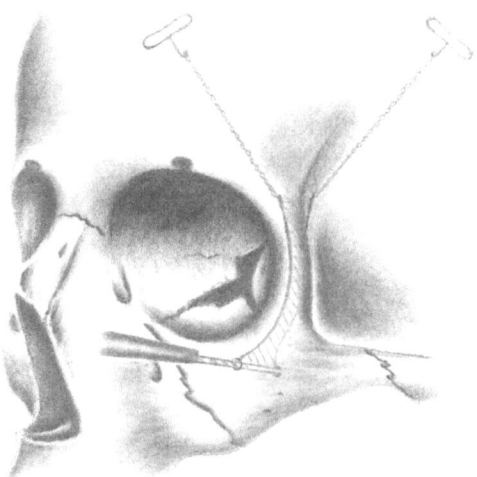

Figure 6–13

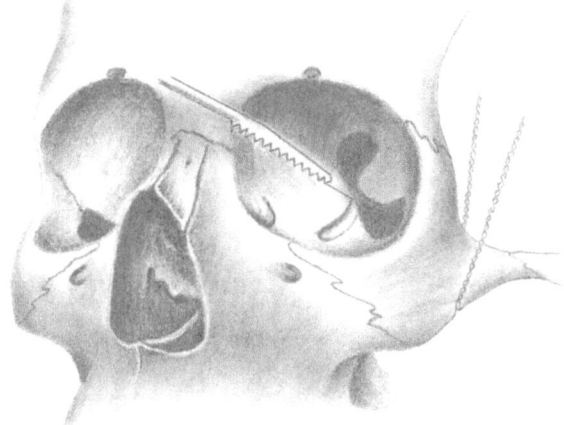

Figure 6–14

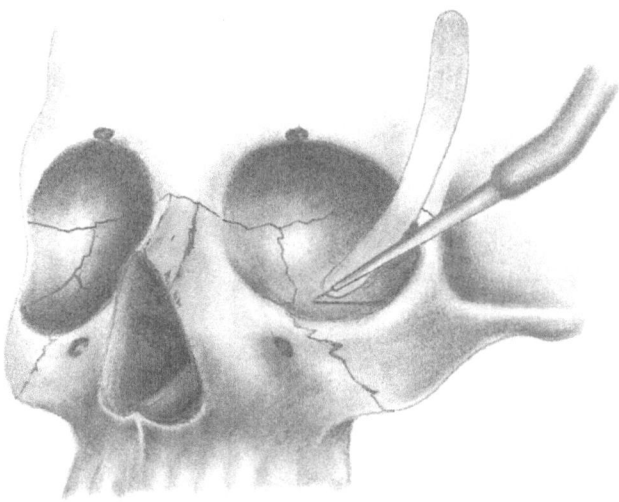

Figure 6–15

Method

The coronal incision is made and the subperiosteal dissection is performed down to the maxillary alveolus and into the orbits. The orbital contents are protected by a malleable retractor. Using a right-angle oscillating saw with a shorter blade, a circumferential osteotomy is made within the bony orbit 1 to 1.5 cm from the orbital rim (Fig. 6-16).

Method

The coronal incision is made and the entire facial soft tissue is separated down to the infraorbital rims subperiosteally. With a malleable retractor, the orbital contents are protected. Using a short, saw-like burr, the osteotomy posterior to the lacrimal apparatus is performed on the lower portion of the medial orbital wall and the medial portion of the orbital floor. The burr should be moved slowly in a seesaw fashion to prevent stalling of the burr and to minimize friction and heat to the bone (Fig. 6-17).

Method

The approach is provided via a coronal incision with subperiosteal dissection down to the temporal fossa. With a malleable retractor, the orbital contents are protected. The osteotomy is performed about 1.5 to 2 cm from the orbital rim in a cephalad direction in the lateral portion of the orbital floor and the lateral orbital wall. Care should be taken to prevent injuring the infraorbital neurovascular bundle (Fig. 6-18).

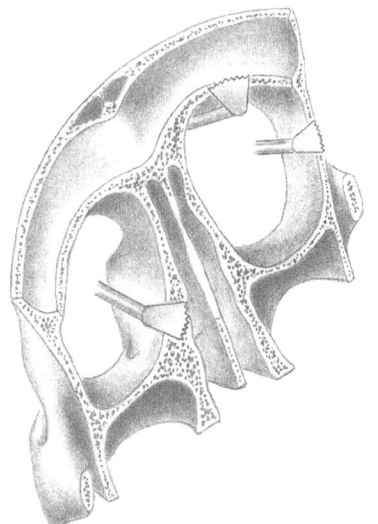

Figure 6–16

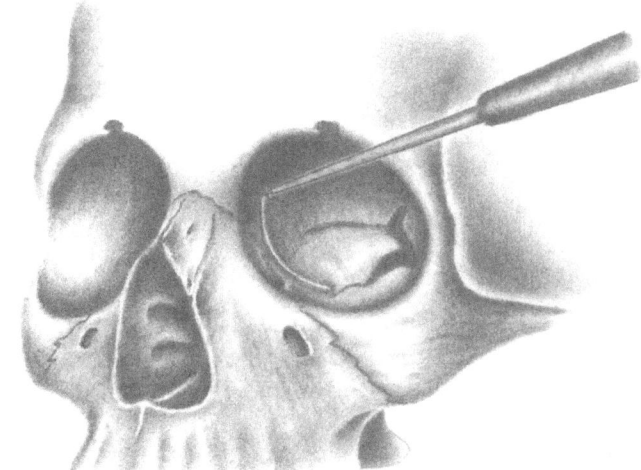

Figure 6–17

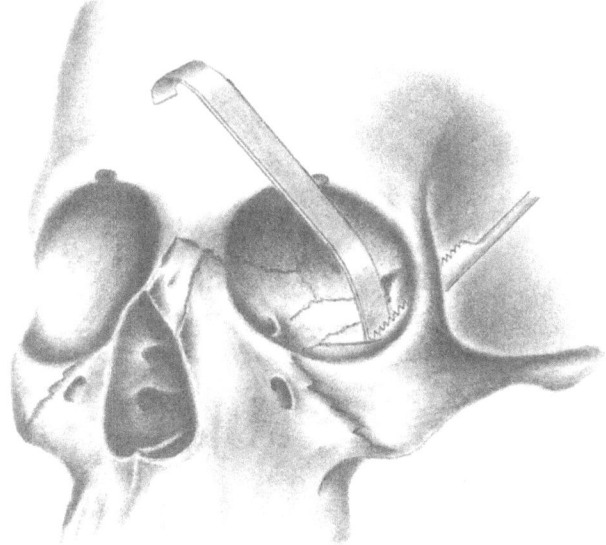

Figure 6–18

Method

The exposure of the frontonasal junction is provided via a coronal incision. With an oscillating saw, the nasal bone is transected just below the cribriform plate. Then a double-ball osteotome is inserted and directed inferior-posteriorly to separate the nasal septum from the cranial base (Fig. 6-19).

Method

After the completion of the craniotomy, a narrow osteotome is placed at the foramen caecum and an osteotomy is made parallel to the nasal bridge on the upper nasal septum. The nasal septum separation at the level of the nasal floor is usually completed by a double-ball osteotome via the upper buccal sulcus incision or the nasal vestibular incision (Fig. 6-20).

Method

After the completion of the craniotomy, the brain is retracted and protected by a malleable retractor. A narrow edge osteotome is placed posteriorly to the crista galli and directed posterior-inferiorly. With gentle taps on the osteotome, the septum is carefully divided from the cranial base (Fig. 6-21).

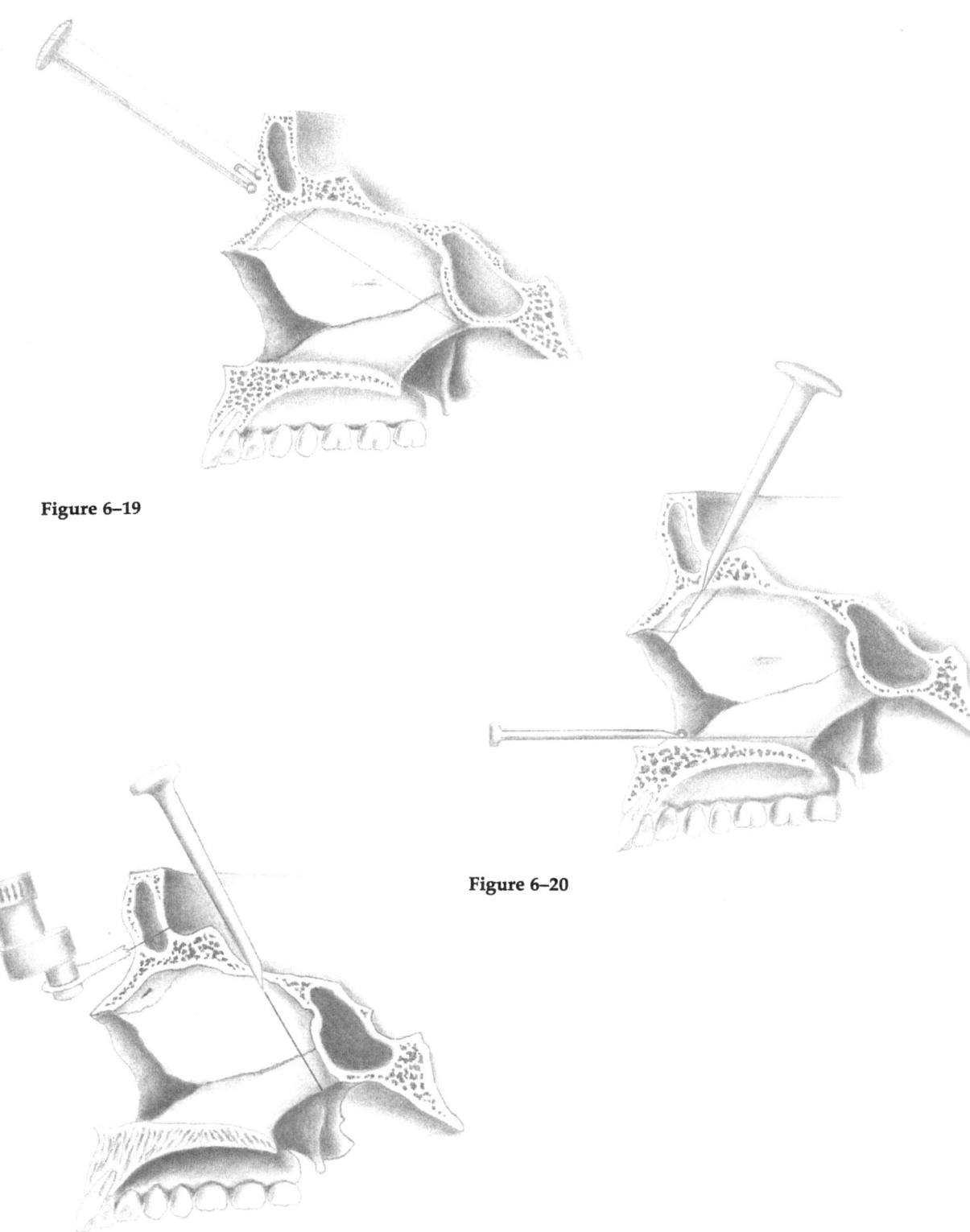

Figure 6–19

Figure 6–20

Figure 6–21

Method

The intranasal intercartilaginous incision is made and subperiosteal dissection is performed over the nasal bone and the paranasal regions. With a hand saw, the osteotomy is made along the base of the bony pyramid. Then a fine curved osteotome is placed at the frontonasal junction. Gentle taps with a hammer will complete the osteotomy (Fig. 6-22).

Method

A mucosa incision is made in the upper oral vestibulum. The periosteum is elevated from the nasal floor and the paranasal regions, leaving the periosteal attachment along the pyriform rim undivided. A reciprocating saw is used to cut the medial wall of the maxilla at the nasal floor. With an osteotome or a right-angle oscillating saw, the paranasal osteotomy is made vertically (Fig. 6-23).

Method

The access to the nasal bone is provided via an intranasal intercartilaginous incision with the periosteum elevated from the nasal bone. A burr with a tissue retractor guard is inserted and moved gently over the nasal arch to remove the excess bone. Heavy pressure against the burr will reduce the speed and cutting efficiency (Fig. 6-24).

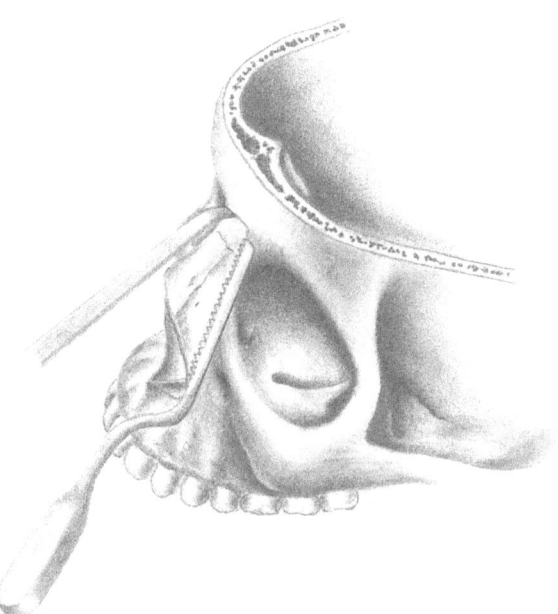

Figure 6–22

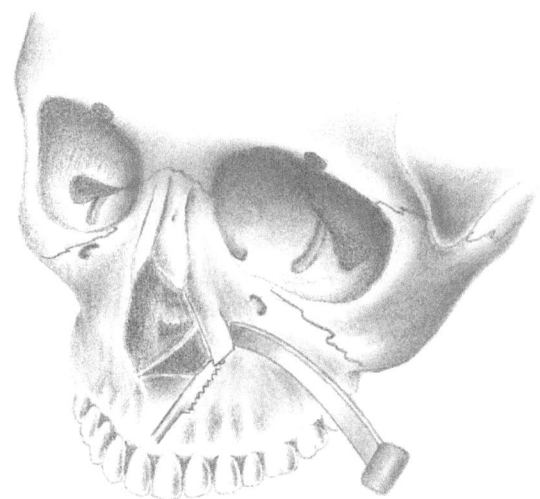

Figure 6–23

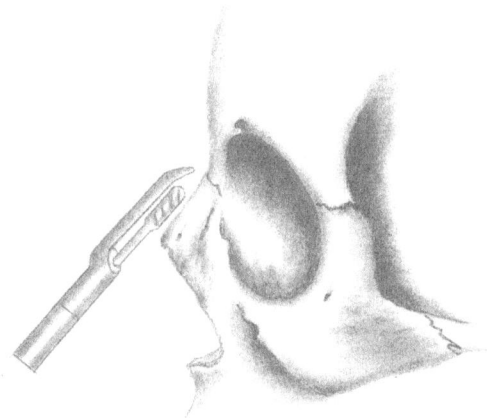

Figure 6–24

Method

Bilateral upper buccal sulcus incisions are made and the subperiosteal dissection is performed over the malar eminence and extended posteriorly to the zygomatic arch. The saw blade is inserted from an inferior-medial to a superior-lateral direction and the two osteotomies are completed on the lateral malar eminence. The middle segment can be removed (Fig. 6-25).

Method

Exposure is provided via the coronal incision and subperiosteal dissection is continued to the nasal bridge and paranasal regions. With a right-angle oscillating saw, the osteotomy is made from the pyriform rim to the infraorbital rim. After the upper buccal sulcus incision is made the osteotomy is performed on the maxillary alveolus between tooth roots by a right-angle oscillating saw (Fig. 6-26).

Method

The coronal incision is used and the subperiosteal dissection is performed down to the maxillary alveolus. The orbital contents are protected by a malleable retractor. With a reciprocating saw, an osteotomy lateral to the nasolacrimal tube is performed sagittally on the frontal maxillary wall and the orbital floor. This can be extended posteriorly to the inferior orbital fissure (Fig. 6-27).

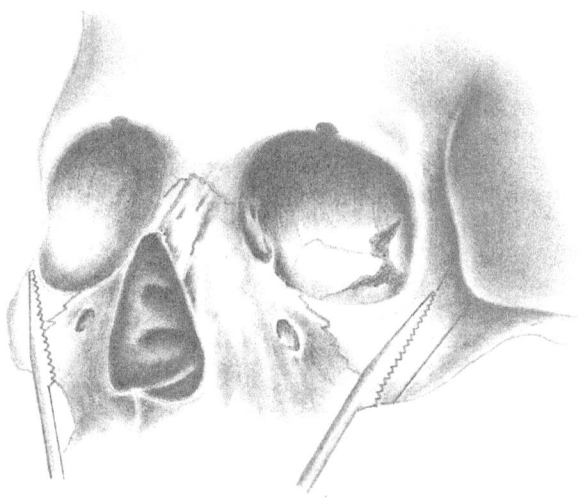

Figure 6–25

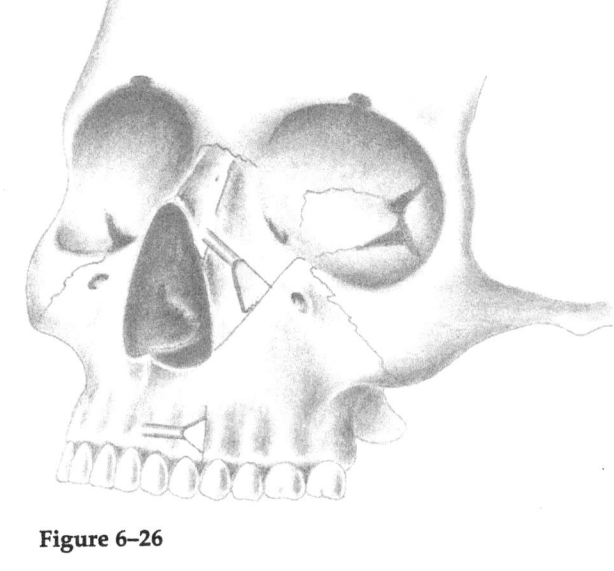

Figure 6–26

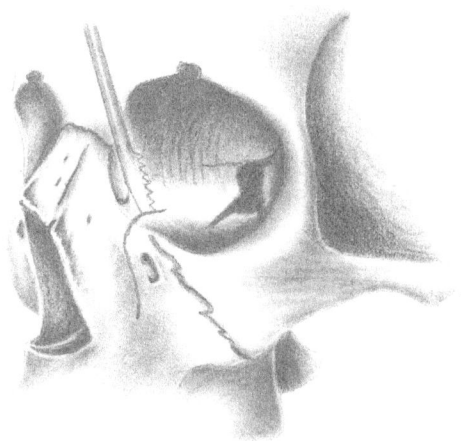

Figure 6–27

Method

The pterygopalatine disjunction can be performed via an intraoral stab wound or via the temporal fossa. The left finger of the surgeon is placed intraorally at the pterygopalatine junction, and the curved osteotome is placed between the pterygoid plate and the maxillary tuberosity. Gentle taps with a hammer by the assistant will complete the separation. During this procedure, the upper edge of the osteotome should be placed away from the maxillary artery and the pterygoid venous plexus (Fig. 6-28).

Method

An upper buccal sulcus incision is utilized and the subperiosteal dissection exposes the maxilla. With a reciprocating saw, the osteotomy is performed horizontally 6 to 8 mm above the dental apices (Fig. 6-29).

Method

An upper buccal sulcus incision is made and the periosteum is elevated from both nasal floors. A fine curved saw is used to cut the posterior portion of the medial maxillary wall (Fig. 6-30).

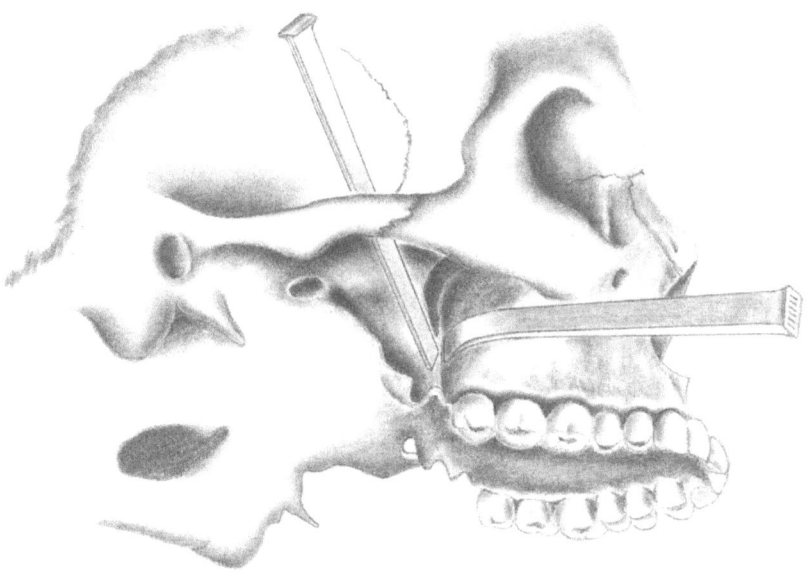

Figure 6–28

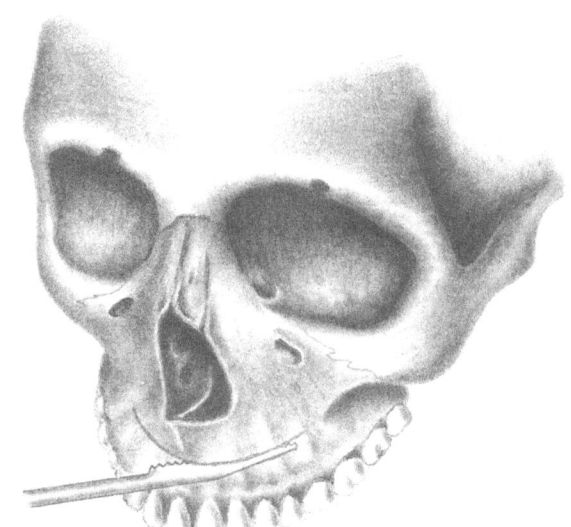

Figure 6–29

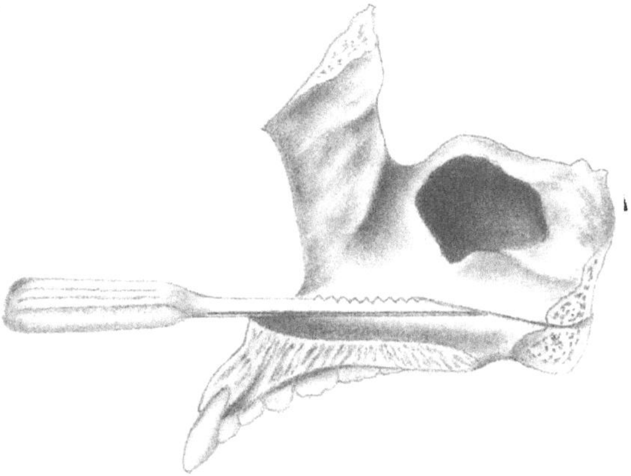

Figure 6–30

Method

The exposure and the horizontal osteotomy proceed in the standard fashion. Then the hole is drilled between the apices, 2 mm above the mandibular canal. A Gigli saw is used to make a vertical cut between the teeth (Fig. 6-31).

Method

Firstly, the lower buccal sulcus incision is made and subperiosteal dissection is completed along the incision. With an oscillating saw, a horizontal osteotomy is performed on the chin at the level 6 mm below the apices. Then the small mucosa incision is made in the medial aspect of the mandible. With a curved elevator, the periosteum is dissected off of the bone. Via the chin osteotomy, a small hand saw is used to cut the medial portions of the both ascending rami (Fig. 6-32).

Method

A vertical mucosa incision is made along the anterior border of the ascending ramus and subperiosteal dissection is carried out as a tunnel to the posterior border of the ramus at the level 2 mm above the mandibular foramen. Using a reciprocating saw, a sagittal osteotomy is made on the ascending ramus through the cancellous bone and extended inferiorly to the predetermined level or the inferior border of the mandible. Care must be taken to prevent injuring the inferior alveolar neurovascular bundle (Fig. 6-33).

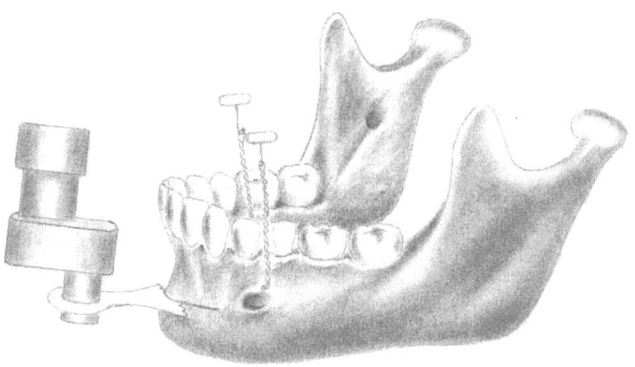

Figure 6–31

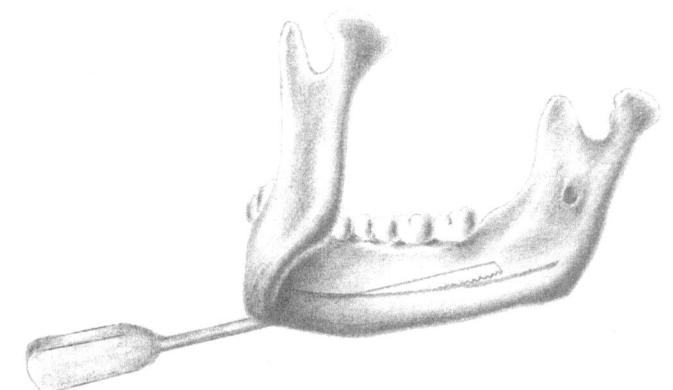

Figure 6–32

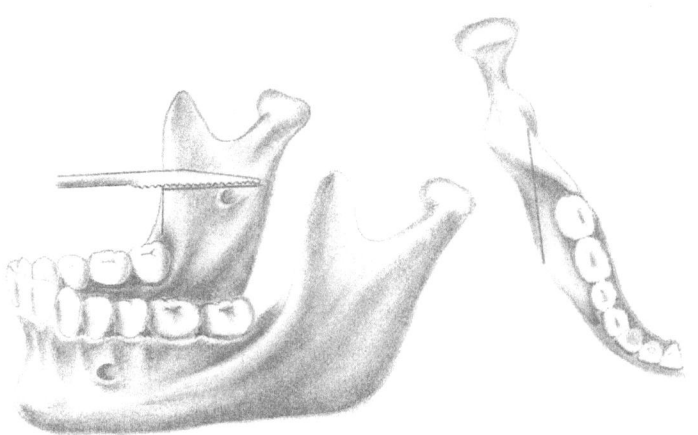

Figure 6–33

Method

A vertical incision is made intraorally along the anterior border of the mandibular ascending ramus. The periosteum is elevated from the lateral or medial aspect of the ramus and continued to the mandibular angle. With a lighted retractor, the important structures medial to the mandibular angle are protected. The osteotomy is carried out by a right-angle oscillating saw with a long shaft and a short blade (Fig. 6-34).

Method

A lower buccal sulcus incision is used for the exposure with subperiosteal dissection made on the mental surface. The bone reduction is completed by an oval burr with irrigation and a tissue retractor guard. Actually, this guard and burr can be used via a small incision while bone is removed in any area where preservation of the overlying soft tissue is mandatory (Fig. 6-35).

Method

This osteotomy is made vertically between the teeth by a small rotary saw with only compact bone cut. Care must be taken to prevent injuring the inferior alveolar neurovascular bundle (Fig. 6-36).

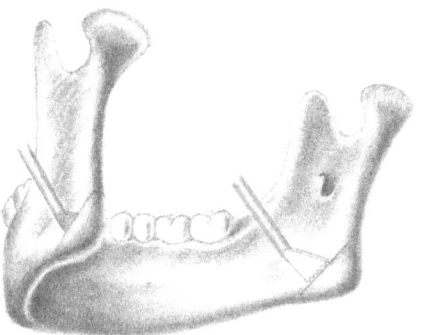

Figure 6–34

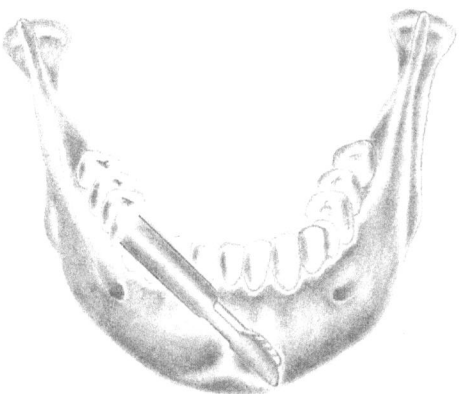

Figure 6–35

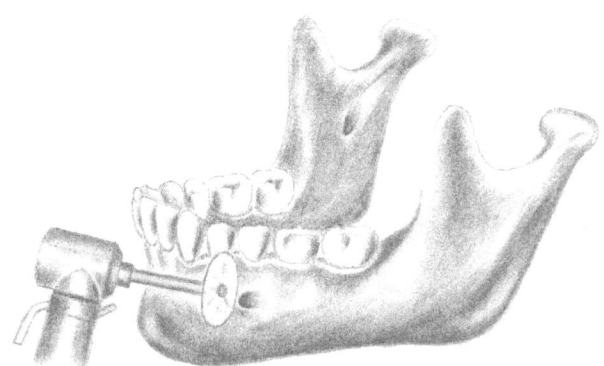

Figure 6–36

Method

The lower buccal sulcus incision is made for the exposure with subperiosteal dissection performed on the mental surface. With a reciprocating saw, the osteotomy is made at the level 6 to 8 mm below the dental apices or 2 to 4 mm below the mental foramen. Care must be taken to prevent injuring the inferior alveolar neurovascular bundle (Fig. 6-37).

Method

A lower buccal sulcus incision is made lateral to the first premolar on either side. Subperiosteal dissection is performed vertically on both ends of the incision. Care must be taken to prevent injuring the mental nerve. By placing the reciprocating saw vertically before the mental foramen, an osteotomy is made around the chin. While the osteotomy is being performed, the left index finger of the surgeon is placed on the inframandibular rim to palpate the saw tip (Fig. 6-38).

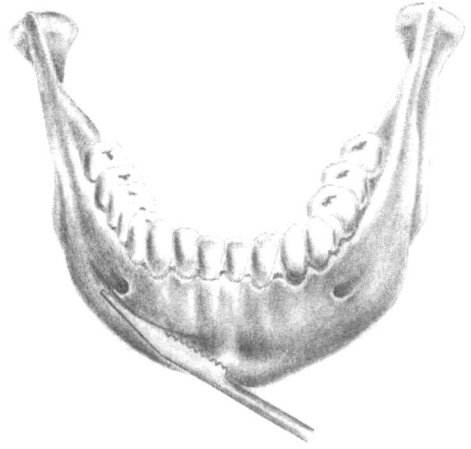

Figure 6–37

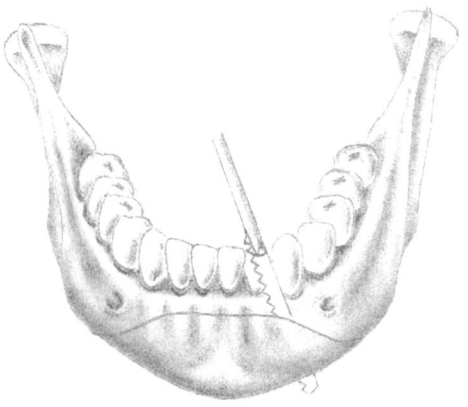

Figure 6–38

Frontal Head

Preoperative Evaluation

On lateral view, the patient shows a retruded upper forehead. Anteriorly, the width of the forehead is normal (Fig. 6-39).

Osteotomy

A standard coronal incision with subperiosteal dissection is made. The craniotomy is performed and the forehead is cut horizontally into several strips. These strips are repositioned to form the desired forehead and rigid fixation is employed (Fig. 6-39).

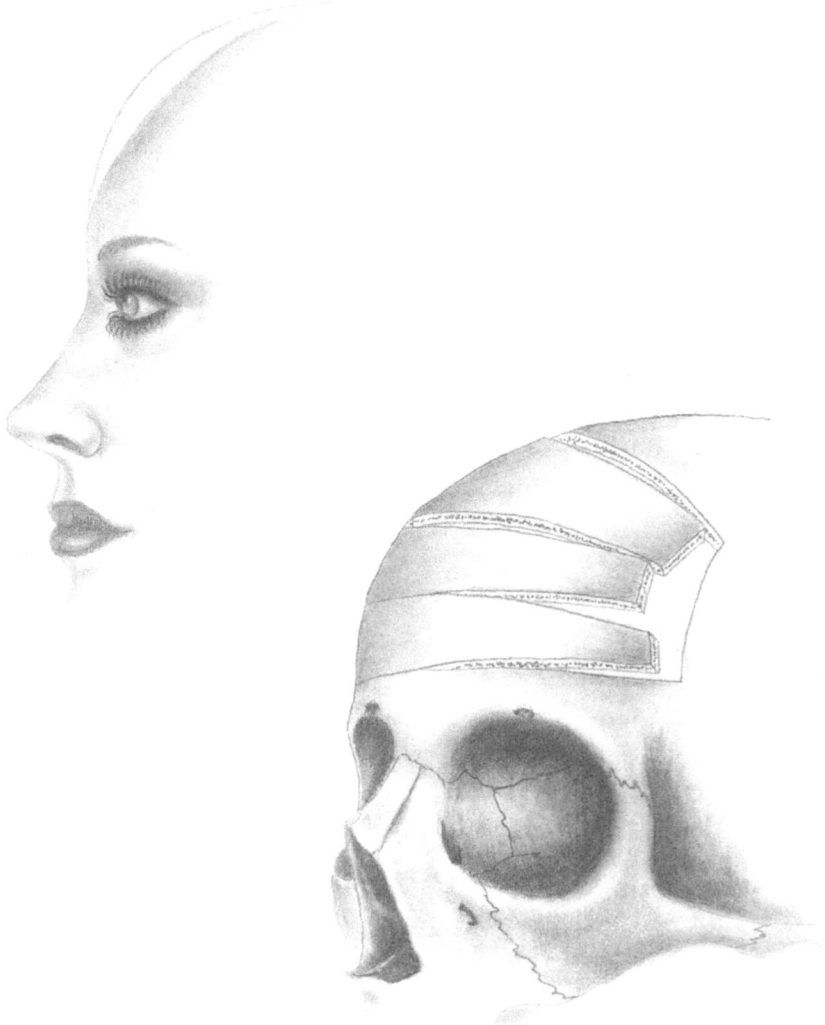

Figure 6–39

Preoperative Evaluation

On basal view, the patient shows a deficiency on both lateral fore-head (Fig. 6-40).

Osteotomy

A coronal incision is made and the periosteum is elevated from the cranial vault and the frontal region. The bone graft for the augmentation is outlined on the cranial vault and cut down to the diploe. With a Gigli saw, the bone grafts are harvested in the manner described previously. The grafts are anchored to the lateral frontal regions with screws (Fig. 6-40).

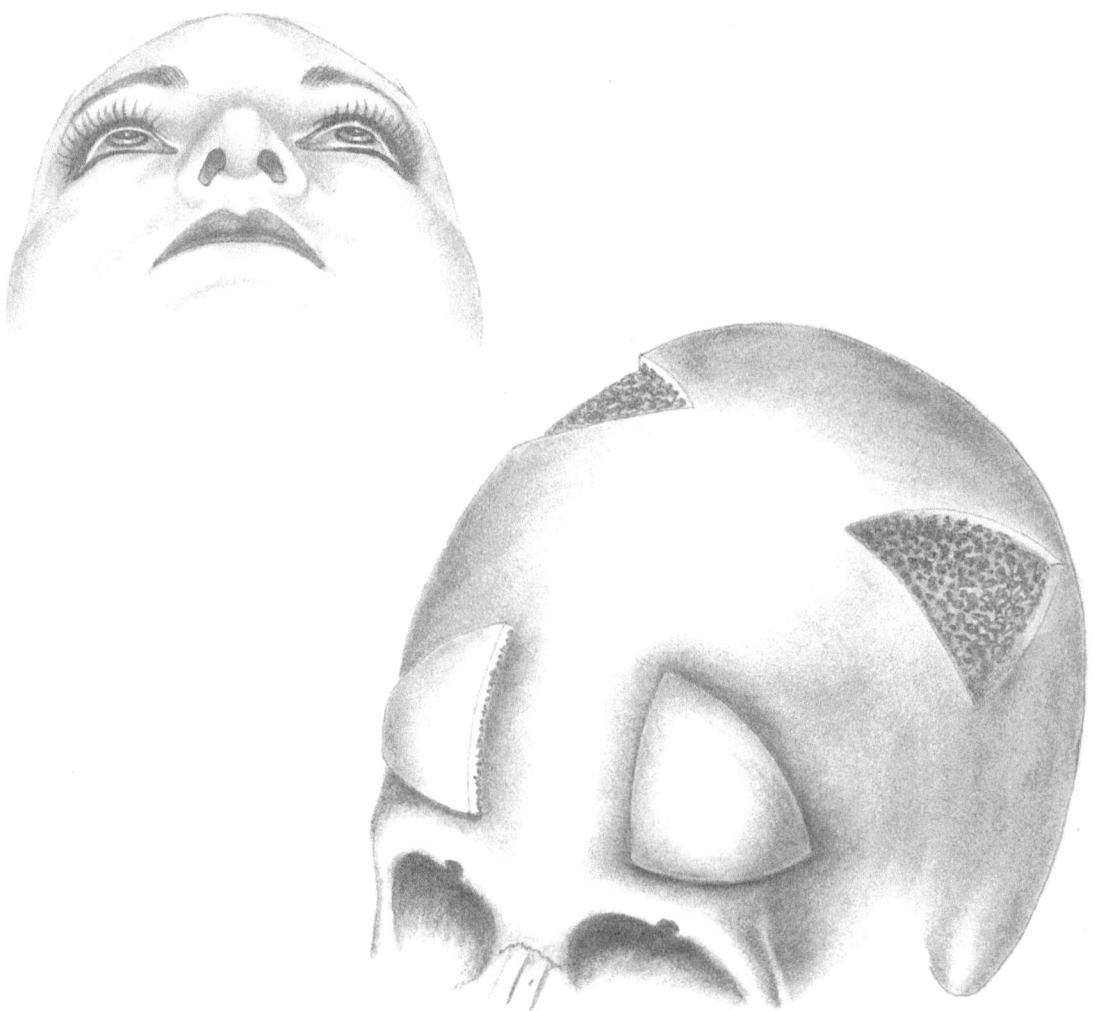

Figure 6–40

Preoperative Evaluation

The patient shows a retruded upper forehead (Fig. 6-41).

Osteotomy

A coronal incision is made and the periosteum is elevated from the forehead. The craniotomy is made 1 cm above the supraorbital rim. The segment is rotated forward and the upper edge is smoothed with a burr. Rigid fixation is used (Fig. 6-41).

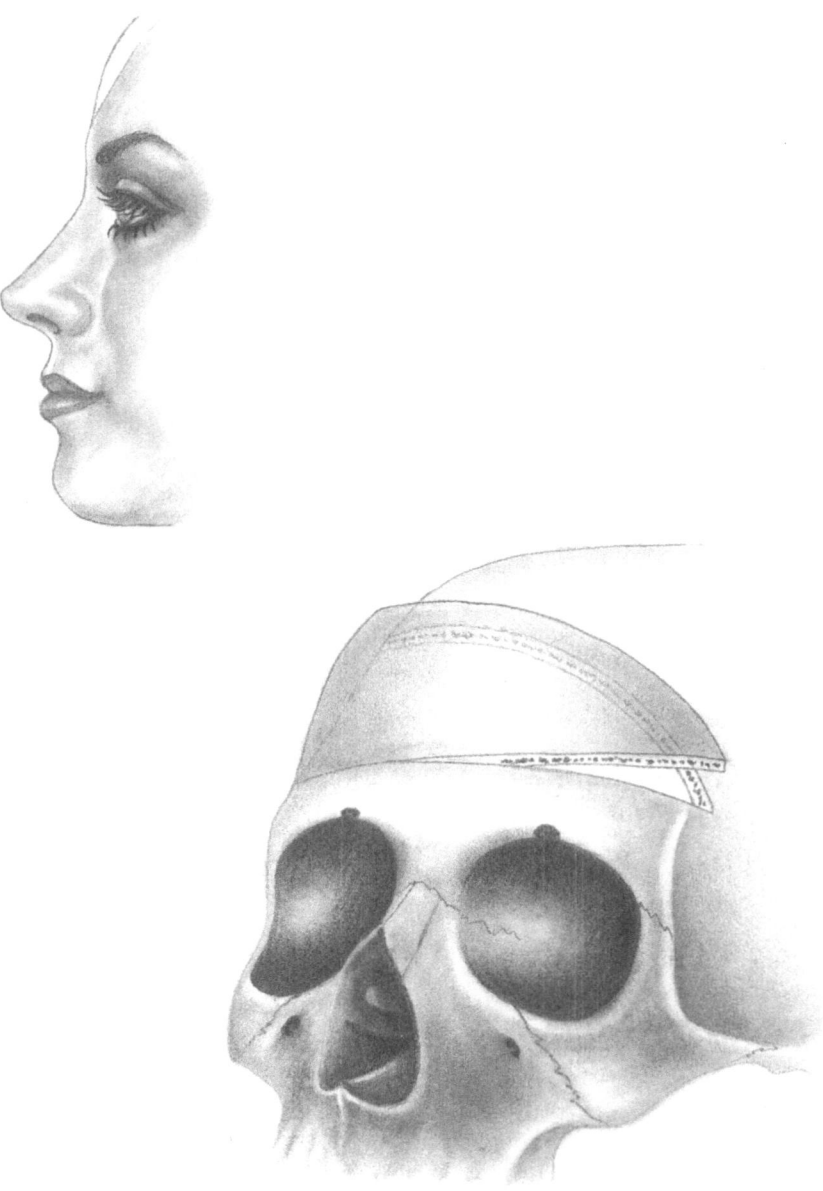

Figure 6–41

Preoperative Evaluation

From basal view, the patient has a narrow upper forehead (Fig. 6-42).

Osteotomy

A standard coronal incision is used. The craniotomy is performed carefully as diagrammed. The desired forehead is selected on the segment and exchanged with the original forehead. Miniplates are employed for the fixation (Fig. 6-42).

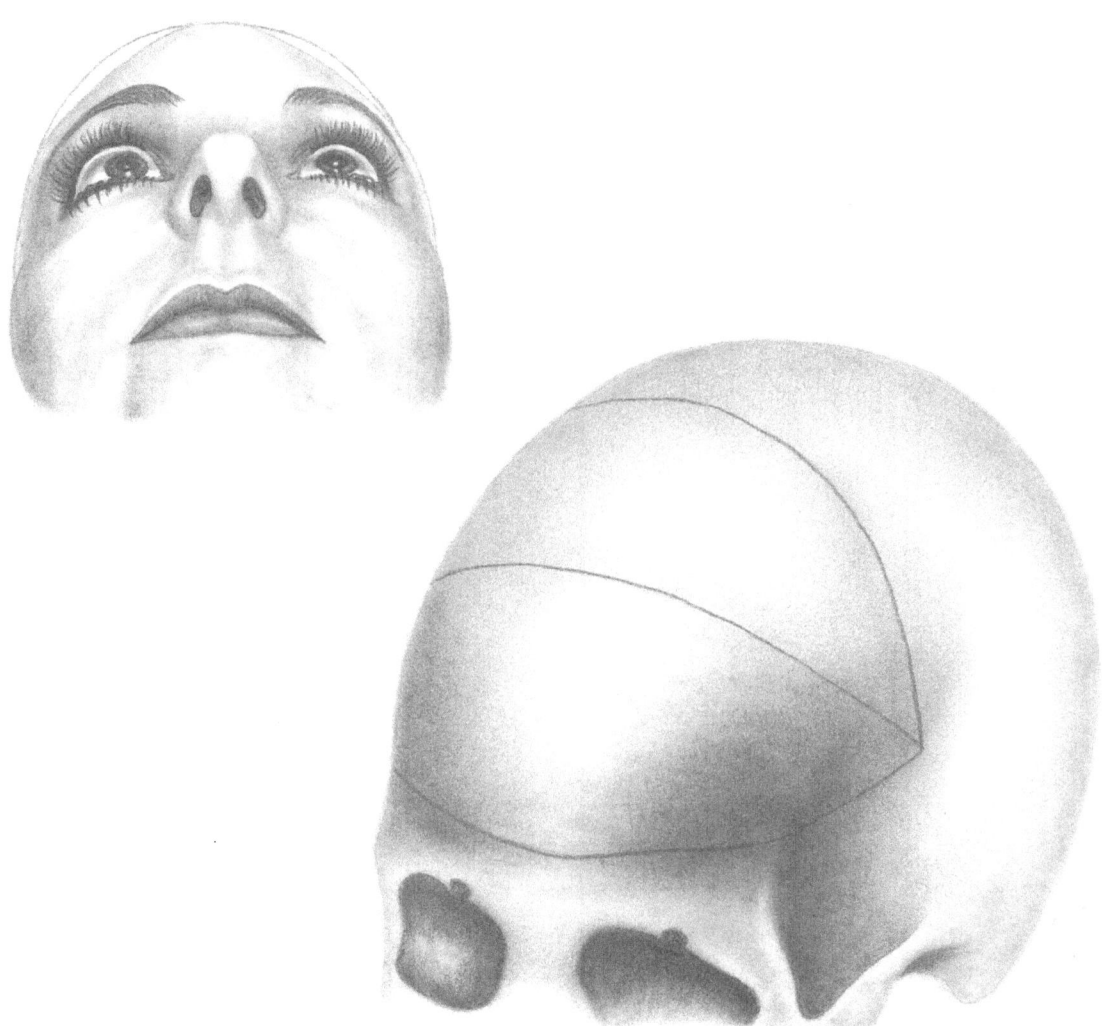

Figure 6–42

Preoperative Evaluation

From lateral view, the patient presents a prominent forehead as well as a flat posterior-cranial vault (Fig. 6-43).

Osteotomy

A coronal incision is made and subperiosteal dissection is carried out over the cranium. A horizontal craniotomy is performed at the level 1 cm above the supraorbital rim. The prominent forehead is cut down as shown. The cranial vault is rotated anterior-inferiorly. Then the forehead bone is repositioned in the posterior-cranium. Rigid fixation is employed (Fig. 6-43).

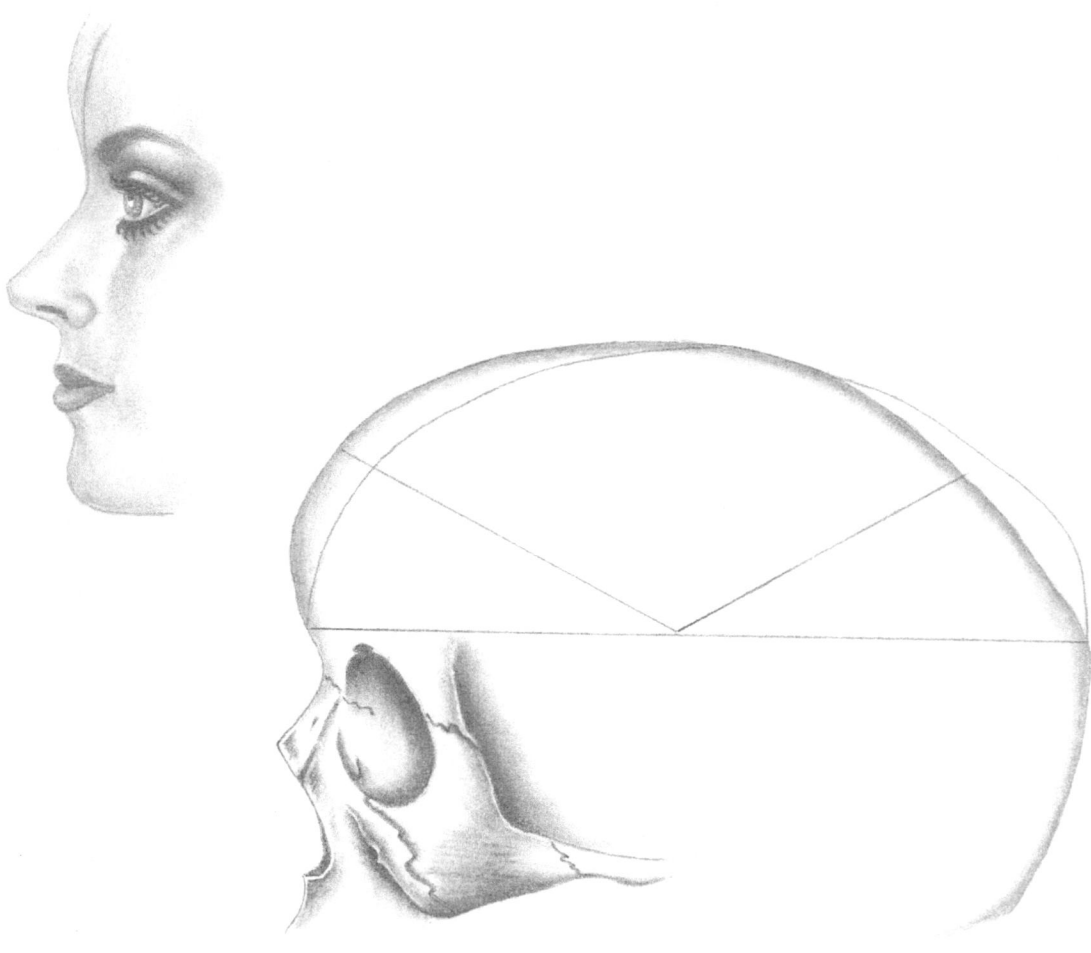

Figure 6–43

Preoperative Evaluation

On lateral view, the patient has a retrusion of the upper forehead with ridging of the supraorbital region (Fig. 6-44).

Osteotomy

A coronal incision is used for exposure and bone graft harvesting. The periosteum is elevated from the upper forehead. Several strips of the cranial outer table are harvested in the manner described previously. The bone grafts are stacked and contoured in the predesign form. Screws are used for the fixation. With an oval burr, the bone graft's edge is smoothed into the surrounding surfaces (Fig. 6-44).

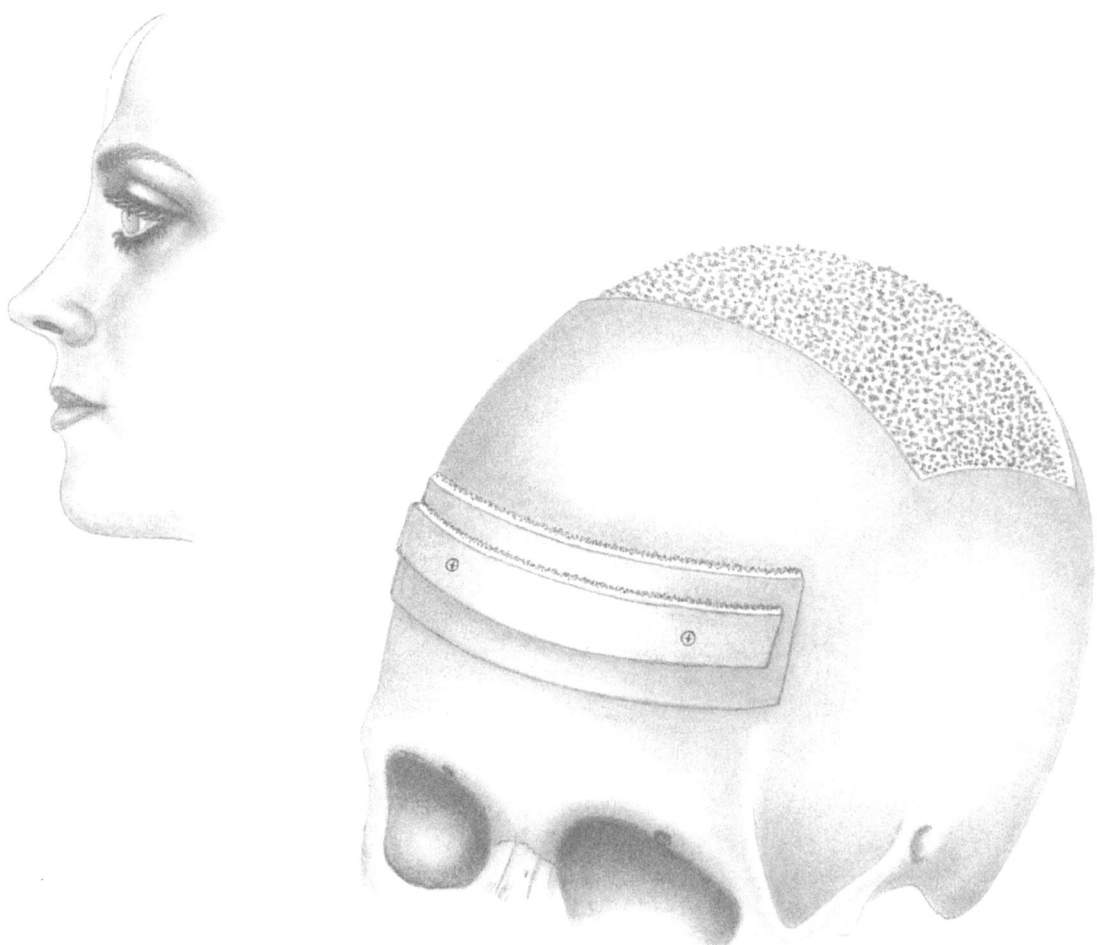

Figure 6–44

Preoperative Evaluation

This patient has a retruded upper forehead as well as a deficiency on the lateral forehead (Fig. 6-45).

Osteotomy

A coronal incision is made and the periosteum is separated from the forehead. The craniotomy is performed 1 cm above the supraorbital rims and the forehead is cut vertically into several curved fans. The forehead is remodeled with these segments. Miniplates and screws are used for the fixation (Fig. 6-45).

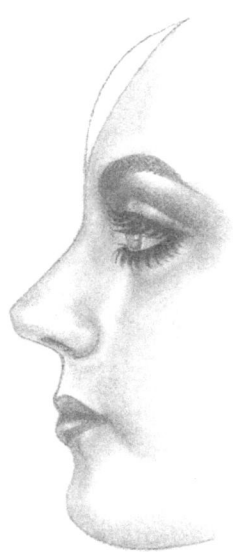

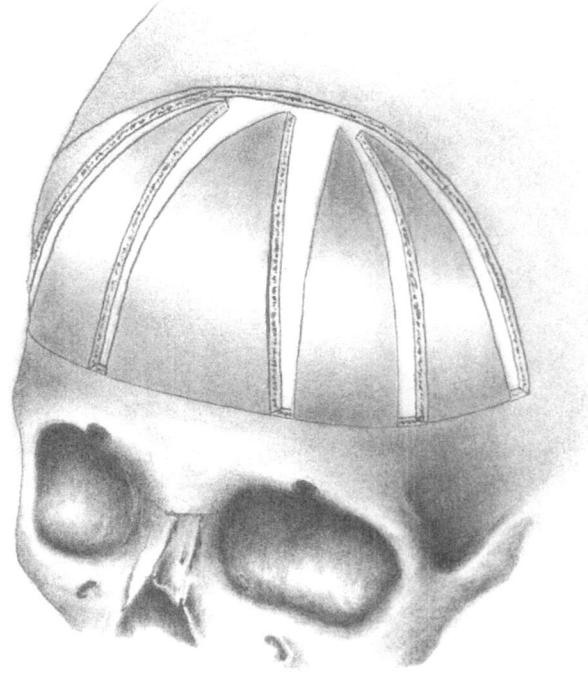

Figure 6–45

Preoperative Evaluation

On basal view, the patient has a narrow and retruded upper forehead (Fig. 6-46).

Osteotomy

A coronal incision is made and subperiosteal dissection is then performed. With a wire pattern, the desired forehead contour is reproduced. This wire pattern is used to select a portion of the calvarium with the proper curvature and outline. With a rotary saw, this outline is cut down to the diploe. A Gigli saw is inserted into the outline and used in seesaw fashion to harvest the outer table. The bone graft is fixed in the upper forehead with screws. The length of the screws should be selected to avoided penetrating the intracranium (Fig. 6-46).

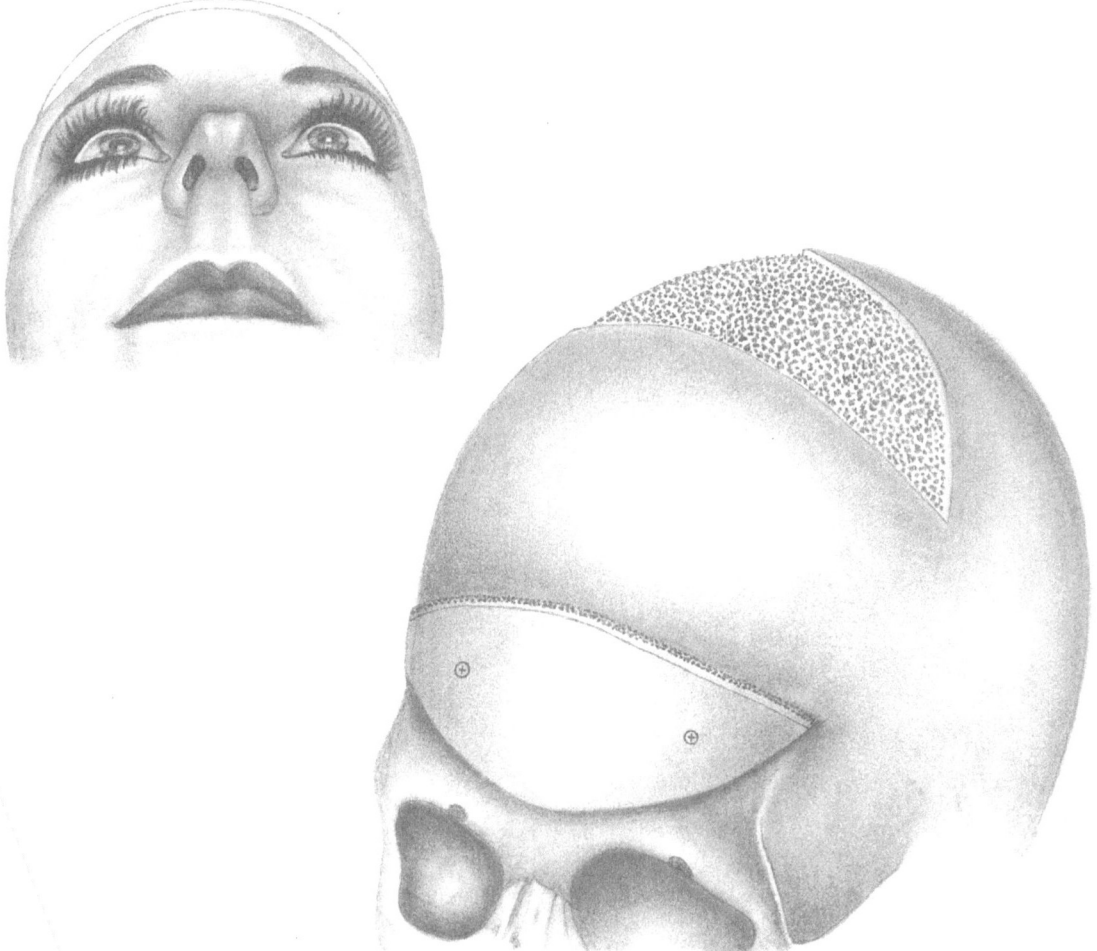

6-46

Preoperative Evaluation

The patient presents a retruded upper face involving forehead, nasal bridge and the lateral orbital rim (Fig. 6-47).

Osteotomy

A coronal incision is made and the subperiosteal dissection is continued to the lateral orbital rims, the nasal bridge, and the paranasal regions. The craniotomy is performed first. With the brain and the orbital contents protected, the osteotomy from within the bony orbit, 1.5 cm from the orbital rim, is made by a right-angle oscillating saw. The lateral orbital rims and the paranasal regions are cut by the oscillating saw as well. The separation of the nasal septum is made from the foramen caecum to the nasal floor by an osteotome. The segment is rotated forward and rigid fixation is employed (Fig. 6-47).

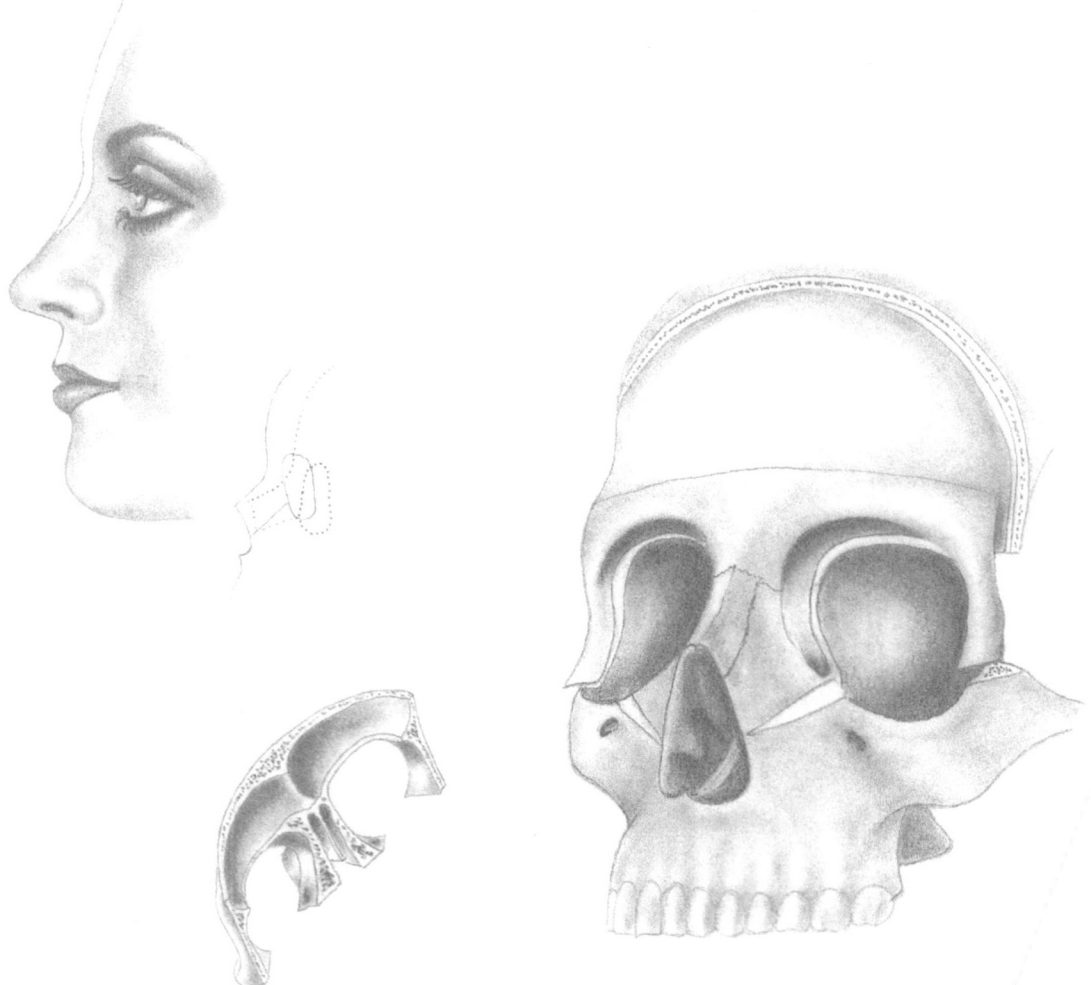

Figure 6–47

Preoperative Evaluation

This patient has a retruded midface involving the orbit, nasal bridge, and the malar eminences. The eyes protrude slightly forward out of the orbital plane. The occlusion is normal (Fig. 6-50).

Osteotomy

The coronal incision and the upper buccal sulcus incision are used for the exposure. Subperiosteal dissection is continued into the orbit, the zygomatic buttress, and the nasal floor. After completion of the craniotomy, the circumferential osteotomy is made within the bony orbit by a right-angle oscillating saw 1.5 cm from the orbital rim. The zygomatic arch and the buttress are cut as shown. An osteotome with a narrow edge is placed at the foramen caecum and the osteotomy is made inferiorly to separate the nasal septum, and the split facial bone is rocked gently by placing an osteotome along the osteotomy lines (Fig. 6-50).

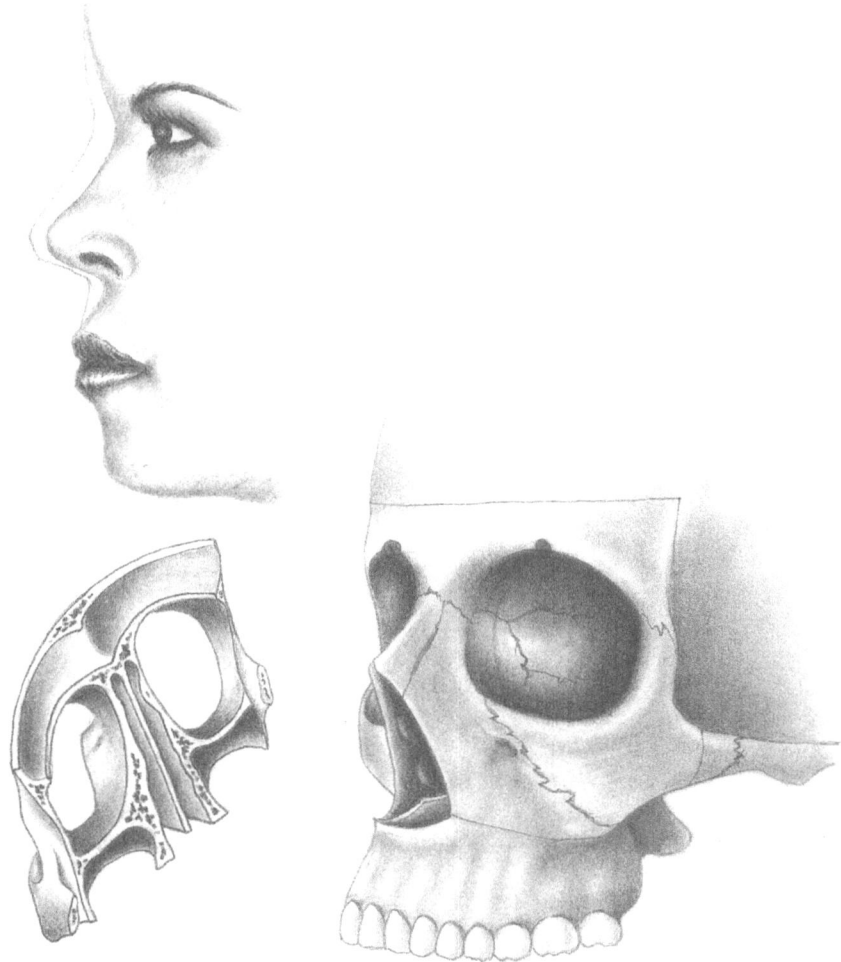

Figure 6–50

Preoperative Evaluation

On side view, this patient presents a slight inclination of forehead, which involves the supraorbital rim (Fig. 6-51).

Osteotomy

A coronal incision is applied and the subperiosteal dissection is continued to the frontal hairline where the advancement of forehead would be made. With an oscillating saw and a curved chisel, the forehead bone is split in situ along the diploic space down to the supraorbital rim. Attention should be paid to the glabellar region. The osteotomy is performed superficially to the frontal sinuses to keep the sinus mucosa intact. Once the osteotomy is finished, the outer table of the forehead bone can be bent forward to the desired position and remodeled into the designed shape. Several pieces of bone grafts in proper thickness are wedged into the gap between the outer table and inner table. No fixation is needed. This technique offers many advantages to craniofacial plastic surgery. It can be applied to most areas on a face to where the thickness of bones is more than 4 mm (Fig. 6-51).

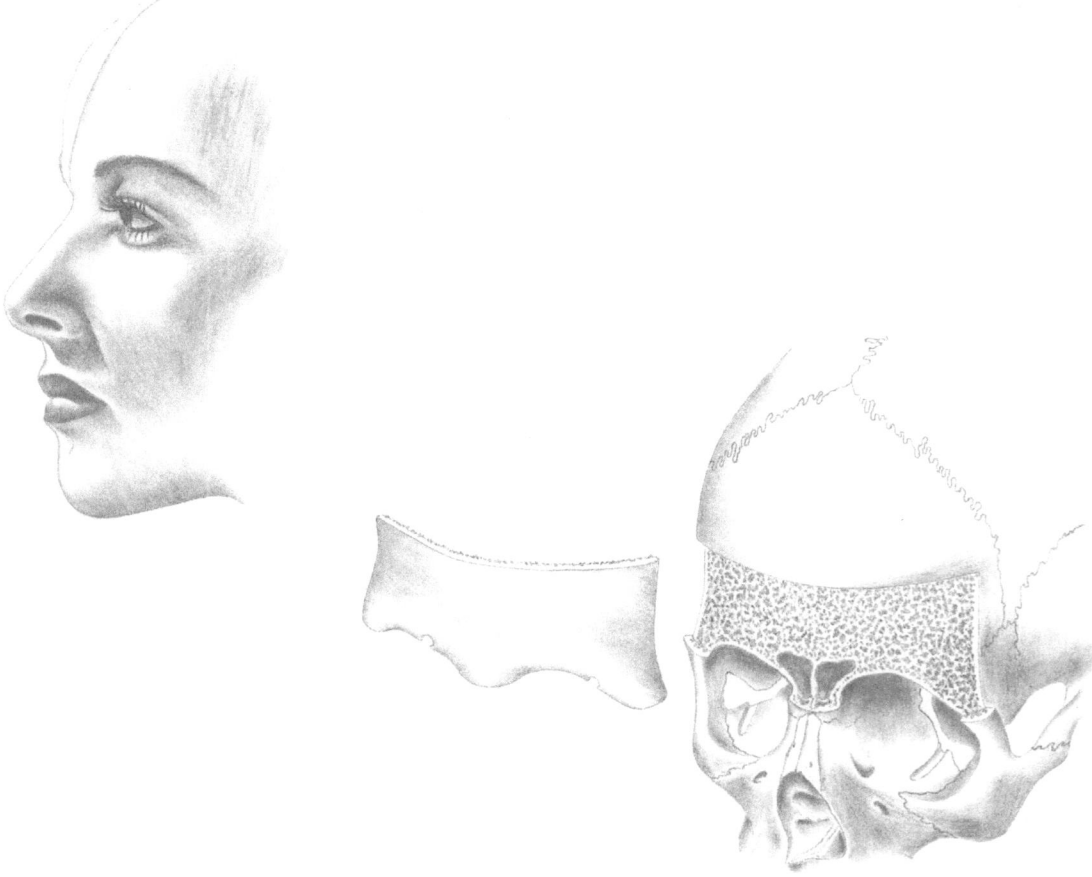

Figure 6–51

Periorbital Region

Preoperative Evaluation

This patient has hypotelorism (Fig. 6-52).

Osteotomy

The exposure is provided via the coronal incision with subperiosteal dissection made down to the infraorbital rims and the temporal fossa. The craniotomy is performed initially. With a reciprocating saw, the posterior-lateral orbital wall is cut. The osteotomy medial to the medial orbital wall is performed sagittally. After all osteotomies are completed, an osteotome is inserted into the osteotomy line to rock the orbit gently until it is entirely mobile. The orbit is moved laterally and miniplate fixation is used (Fig. 6-52).

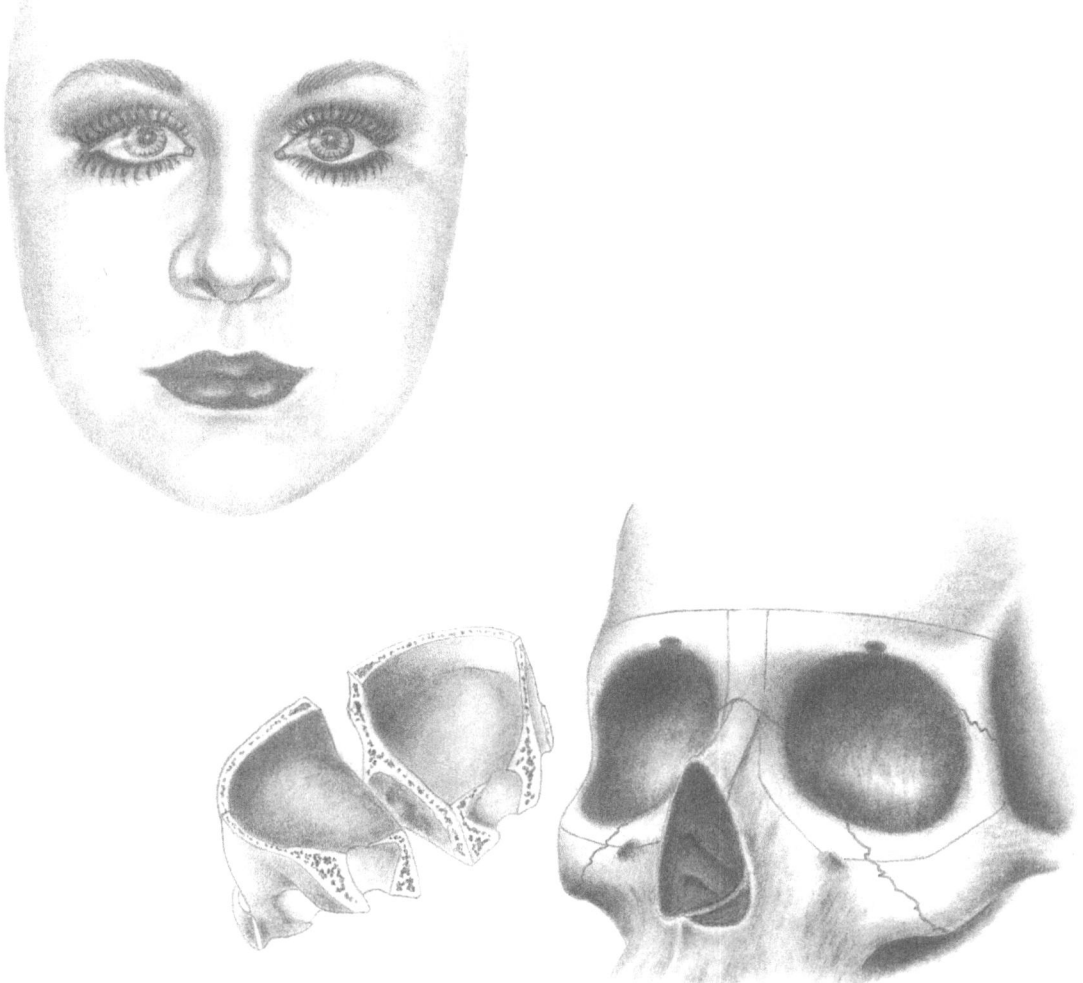

Figure 6–52

Preoperative Evaluation

On three-quarter view, the patient shows marked prominence of the superior-lateral orbital ridges (Fig. 6-53).

Osteotomy

The coronal, the upper blepharoplasty, or the infrabrow incision can be used for the exposure. The subperiosteal dissection is carried out over the superior-lateral orbital region. Using a small reciprocating saw and an oval burr with a guard, the bony prominence is reduced until the desired result is obtained. The orbital rim periosteum is sutured into an expanded position. This is important to prevent the ptotic brow. Overcorrection should be avoided (Fig. 6-53).

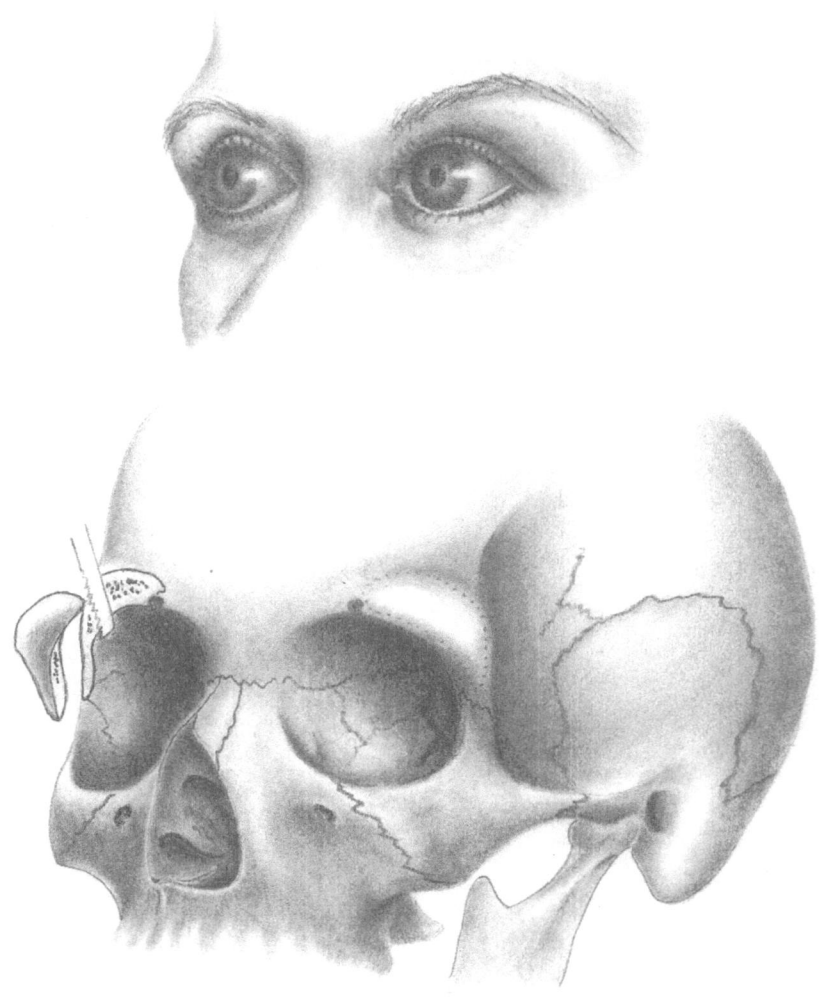

Figure 6–53

Preoperative Evaluation

The patient has an excessive prominence of the glabella and the area of the frontal sinus (Fig. 6-54).

Osteotomy

The coronal incision, the upper blepharoplasty incision, or the intrabrow incision can be used for the treatment of this deformity, depending on the degree of the deformity. If the prominence is moderate and the anterior frontal sinus wall is thick enough so that when the reduction is completed the frontal sinus will not be exposed, the osteotomy is performed by an oval burr with a guard via a small infrabrow incision. Care must be taken to protect the frontal nerve. If the reduction involves all of the anterior frontal sinus wall, the exposure is provided via a coronal incision. The osteotomy parallel to the frontal head is carried out with a reciprocating saw. Then the frontal segment is contoured and replaced to the opening on the frontal sinus wall and wires are used for fixation (Fig. 6-54).

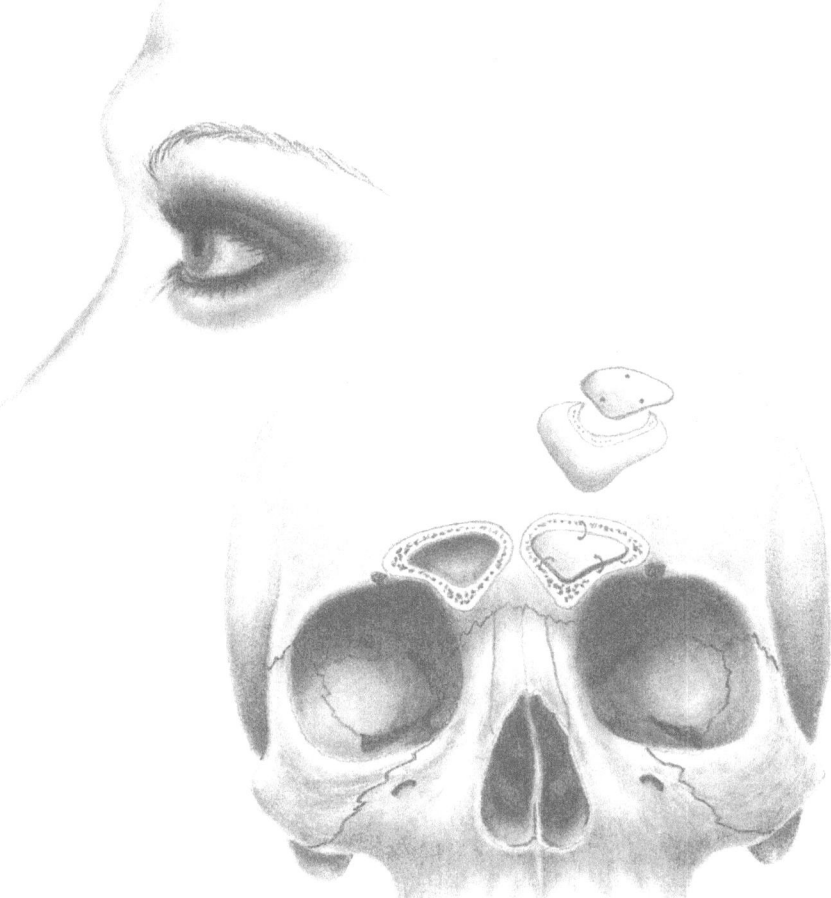

Figure 6–54

Preoperative Evaluation

The patient has hypotelorism (Fig. 6-55).

Osteotomy

The coronal incision with subperiosteal dissection is performed down to the infraorbital rims and continued along the medial and the lateral orbital walls. After the craniotomy, the osteotomies are made with the brain and the orbital contents protected. Using a right-angle oscillating saw with a short blade, a circumferential osteotomy is made within the bony orbit. The frontal osteotomy is completed on both sides. Then an osteotome is placed along the osteotomy and rocked until the entire bony orbit is mobile. The orbit is moved laterally to the new position and rigid fixation is employed. During this procedure, the medial and the lateral canthal tendons must be left attached (Fig. 6-55).

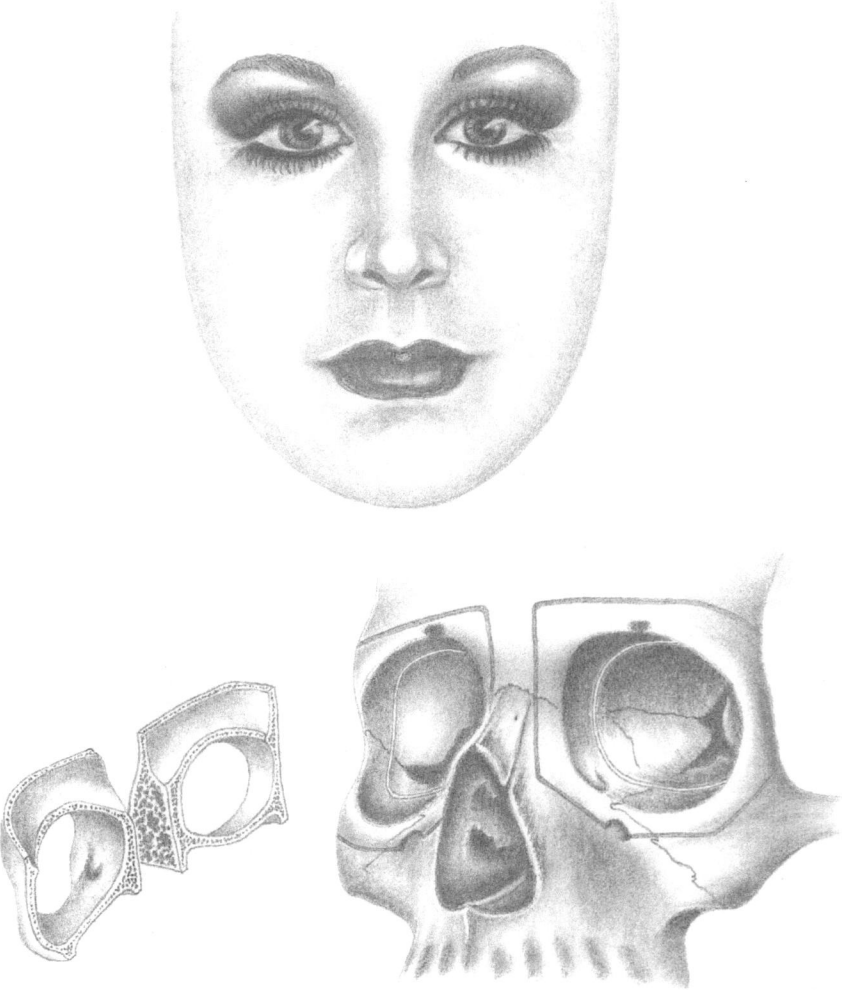

Figure 6–55

Preoperative Evaluation

The patient shows orbital rim infringement in the superior-lateral orbit, which is usually confused with the skin ptosis of the same area (Fig. 6-56).

Osteotomy

The exposure is provided via the upper blepharoplasty incision or the coronal route. Subperiosteal dissection is made along the superior-lateral orbital rim. The infringed bone is removed by an oval burr with a guard or a reciprocating saw as shown. Care must be taken to prevent injuring the supraorbital nerve (Fig. 6-56).

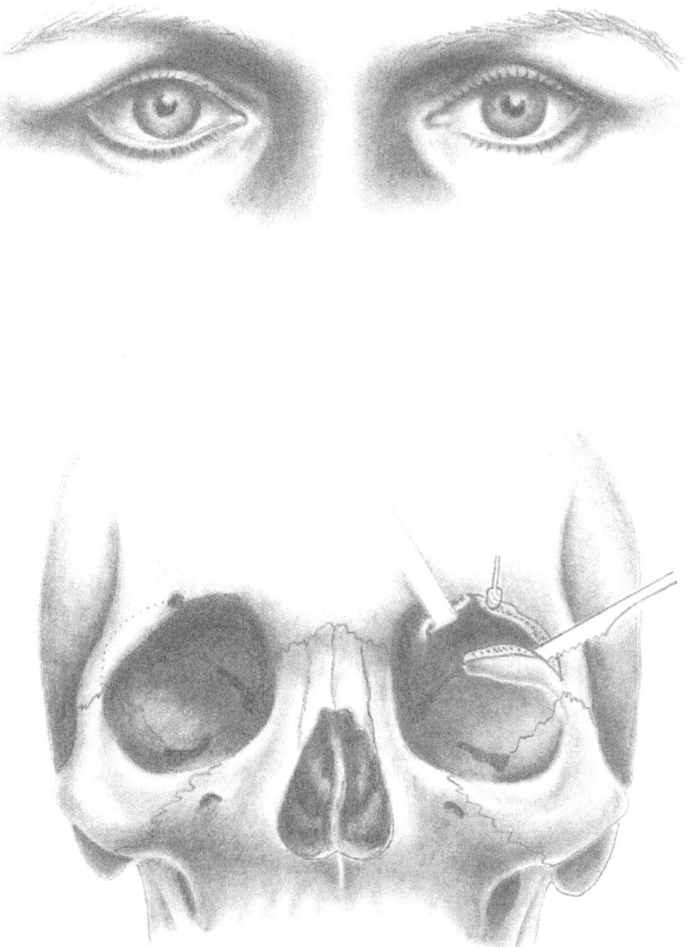

Figure 6–56

Preoperative Evaluation

The patient has a droop in the inferior-lateral orbital rim, but the lateral canthal tendon is attached at the normal position (Fig. 6-57).

Osteotomy

Exposure is provided via the lower blepharoplasty incision and the periosteum is elevated from the orbital floor. The bone graft is harvested from the cranium. After contouring, the bone graft is placed on the orbital floor and wires are used for fixation (Fig. 6-57).

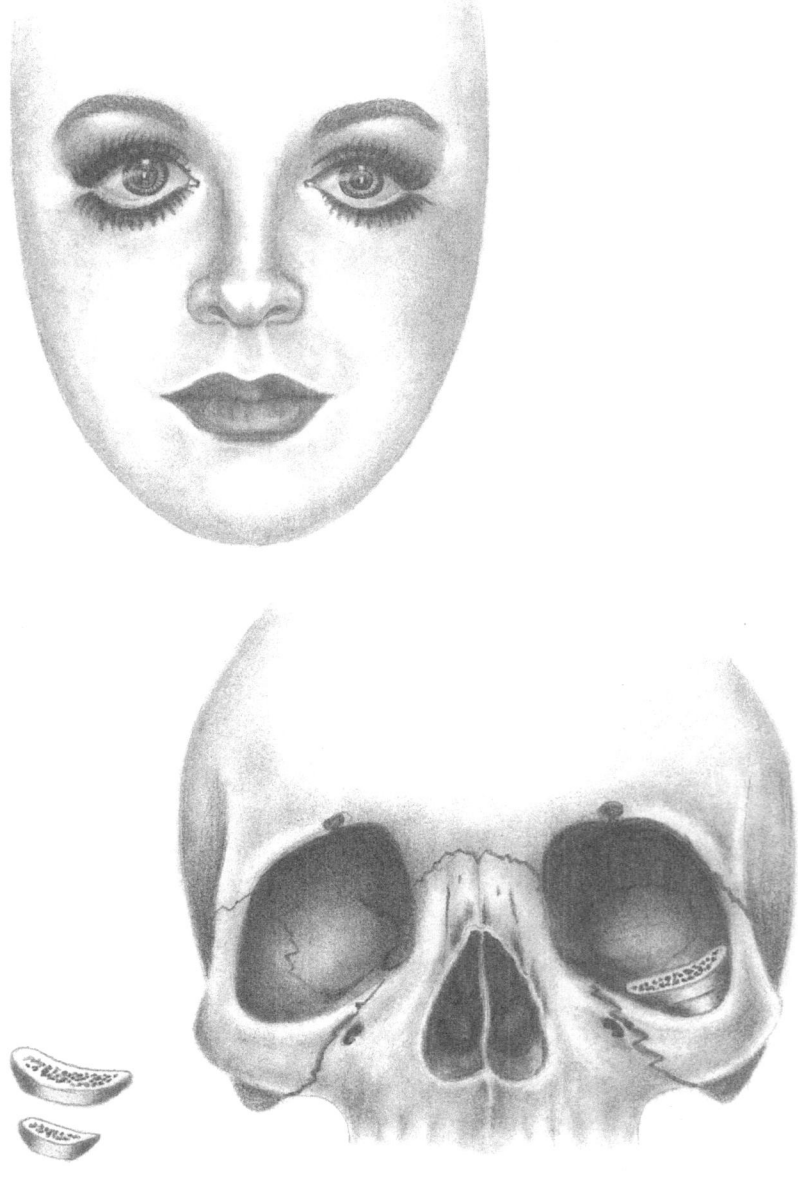

Figure 6–57

Preoperative Evaluation

The patient demonstrates lateral canthal droop involving the inferior-lateral orbital rims (Fig. 6-58).

Osteotomy

A coronal incision is used for the exposure, and subperiosteal dissection is performed over the lateral orbital rims and the frontal portion of the temporal fossa. With a right-angle oscillating saw, the inferior orbital rim is cut. With the orbital contents protected, the lateral orbital wall is cut behind the lateral canthal tendon attachment by a reciprocating saw via the temporal fossa. Once these osteotomies are completed, the segment is moved cephalad. Several screws are used for fixation. An oval burr is used to smooth the segment edge (Fig. 6-58).

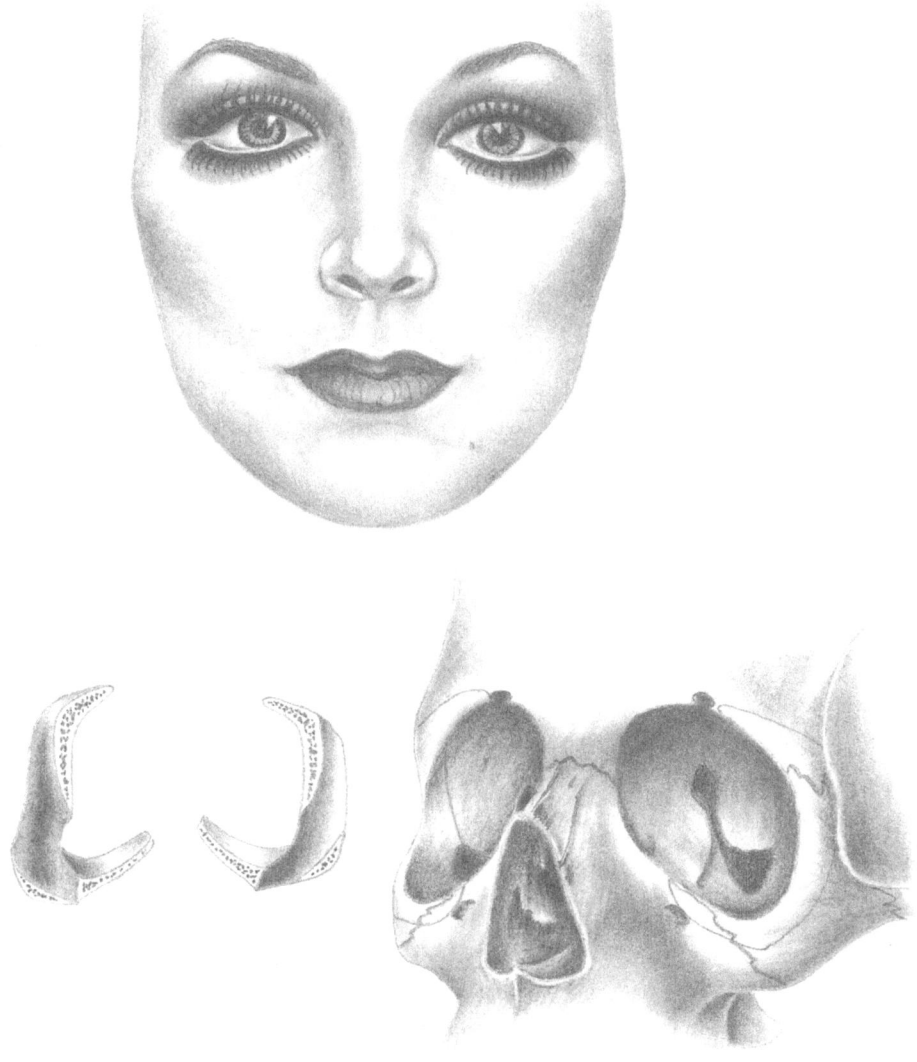

Figure 6–58

Preoperative Evaluation

On lateral view, the patient demonstrates exophthalmos (Fig. 6-59).

Osteotomy

The frontal hairline incision is made bilaterally. Subperiosteal dissection is made on the lateral orbital rim. With a reciprocating saw, the osteotomy is made on the lateral orbital wall anteriorly to where the lateral canthus attaches. The segment is moved forward and the bone graft is inserted in the gap. Rigid fixation is employed (Fig 6-59).

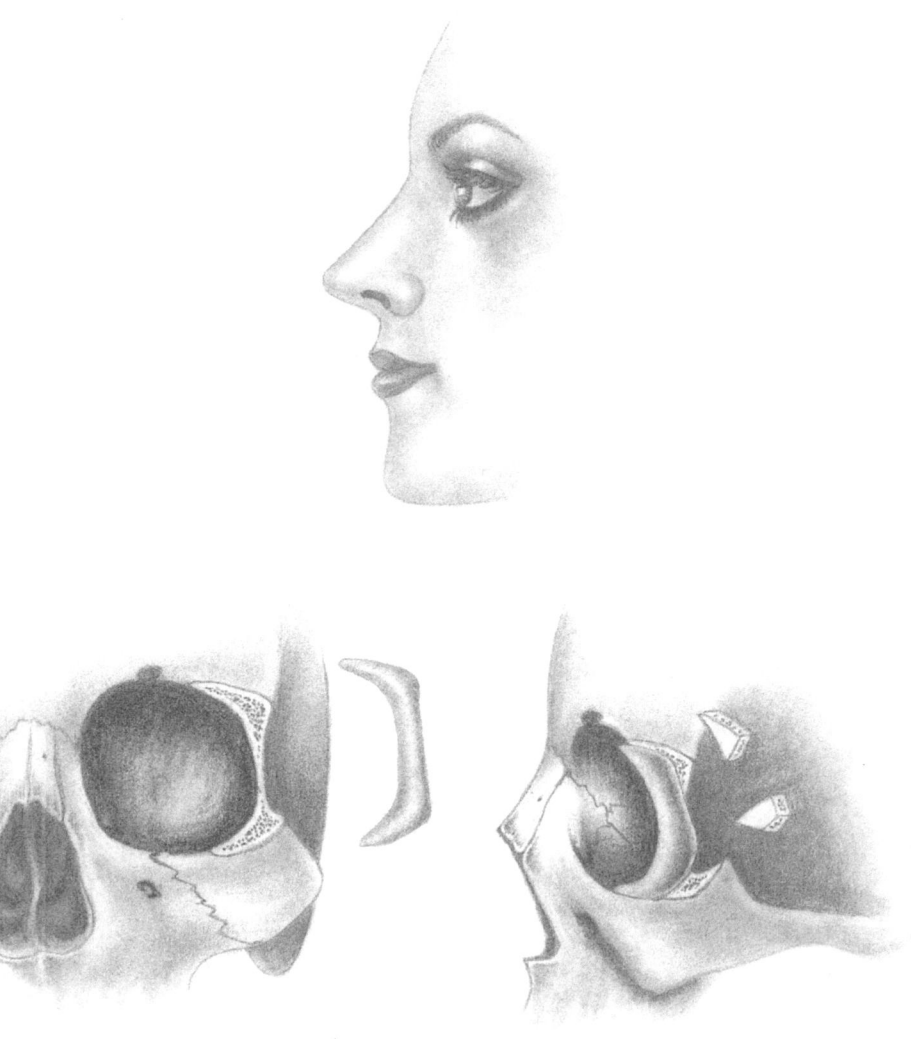

Figure 6–59

Preoperative Evaluation

This patient presents a narrow palpebral fissure width as shown on the right side (Fig. 6-60). (Persons who are Chinese, Korean, or Japanese are among those who may present a narrow palpebral fissure width.)

Osteotomy

The lower blepharoplasty incision is made and the lateral orbital rim is exposed. The lateral canthus must be left attached and undisturbed. With a right-angle oscillating saw and a small osteotome, the lateral orbital rim including the lateral canthus attachment is cut and moved medially. Screw fixation is employed and asymmetry should be avoided (Fig. 6-60).

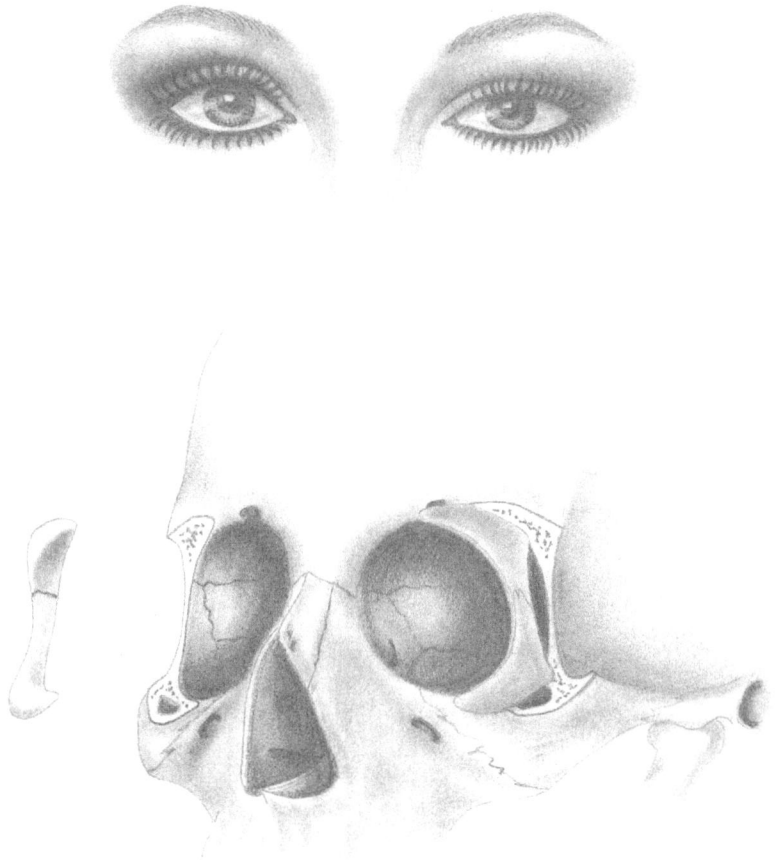

Figure 6–60

Preoperative Evaluation

The patient has hypertelorism (Fig. 6-61).

Osteotomy

The coronal incision is made and subperiosteal dissection is performed down to the infraorbital rims and the temporal fossa. The craniotomy is performed first. With a reciprocating saw, the posterior-lateral orbital wall is cut followed by two parallel sagittal osteotomies at the distance desired. These are made medial to the medial orbital wall. A right-angle oscillating saw with a short blade is used to make an osteotomy 5 mm below the inferior orbital rim. These procedures are repeated on the contralateral side. The orbits are rocked gently until they are entirely mobile and moved medially. Miniplates fixation is used (Fig. 6-61).

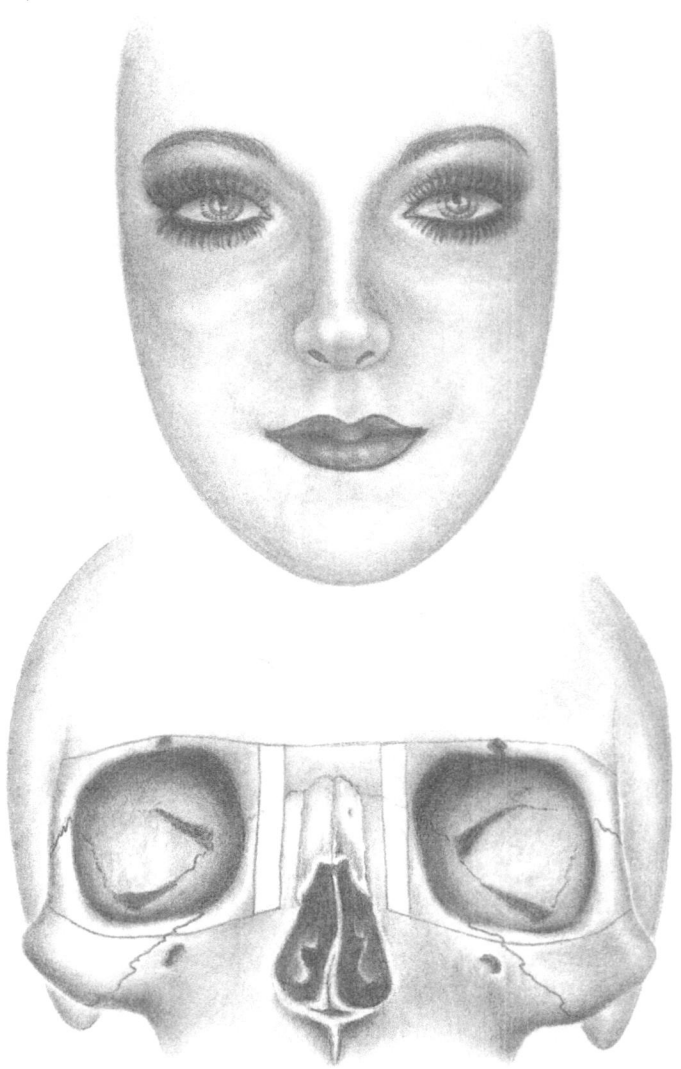

Figure 6–61

Nasal Region

Preoperative Evaluation

The patient has a wide nasal base and a retrusion at the subnasal region (Fig. 6-62).

Osteotomy

An upper buccal sulcus incision is made and the periosteum is separated from the subnasal, paranasal regions, and the nasal floor. With an oscillating saw, a horizontal osteotomy is made at the subnasal region 6 mm above the dental apices. Then an oblique osteotomy is made on both nasal floors and the nasal septum is separated by a double-ball osteotome. Finally, the paranasal osteotomies are completed. The middle segment is moved forward and the lateral segments are pushed medially. Rigid fixation is employed for stabilization of the lateral segments (Fig. 6-62).

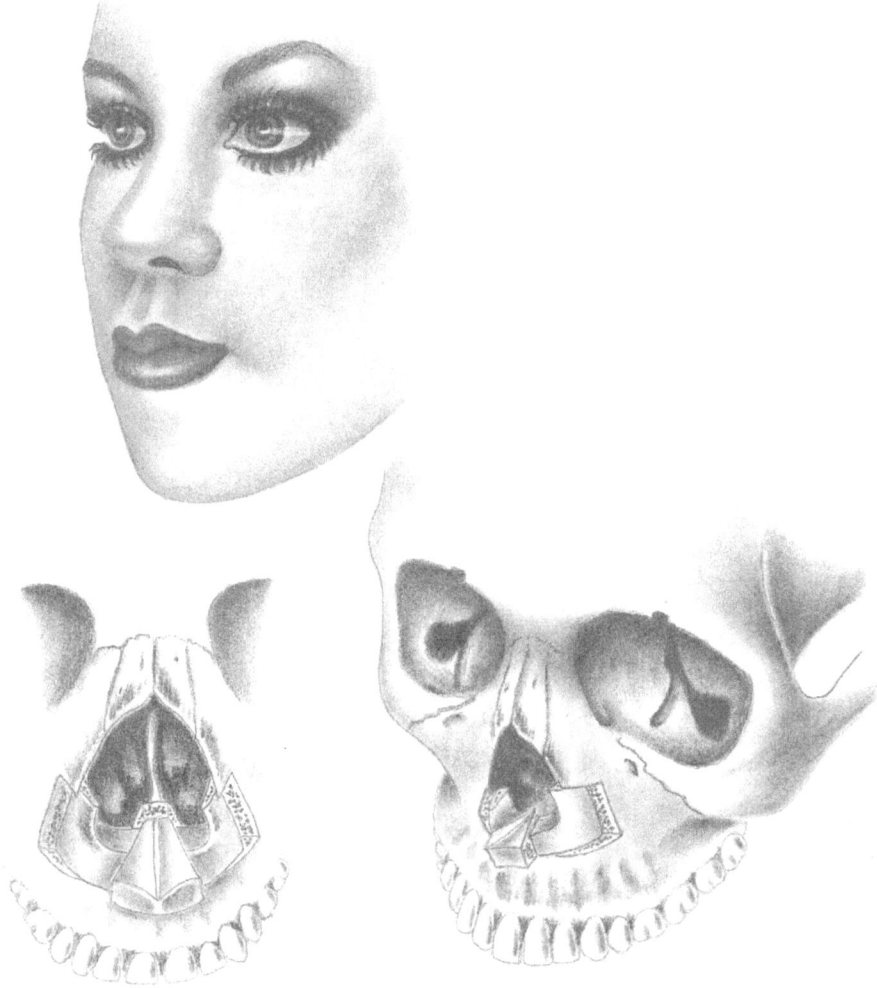

Figure 6–62

Preoperative Evaluation

On basal view, the patient has a wide nasal base and nares (Fig. 6-63).

Osteotomy

Exposure is provided via an upper buccal sulcus incision and the periosteum is elevated from the paranasal region. With an oscillating saw, the osteotomies are performed as shown. The segments are pushed medially and rigid fixation is employed (Fig. 6-63).

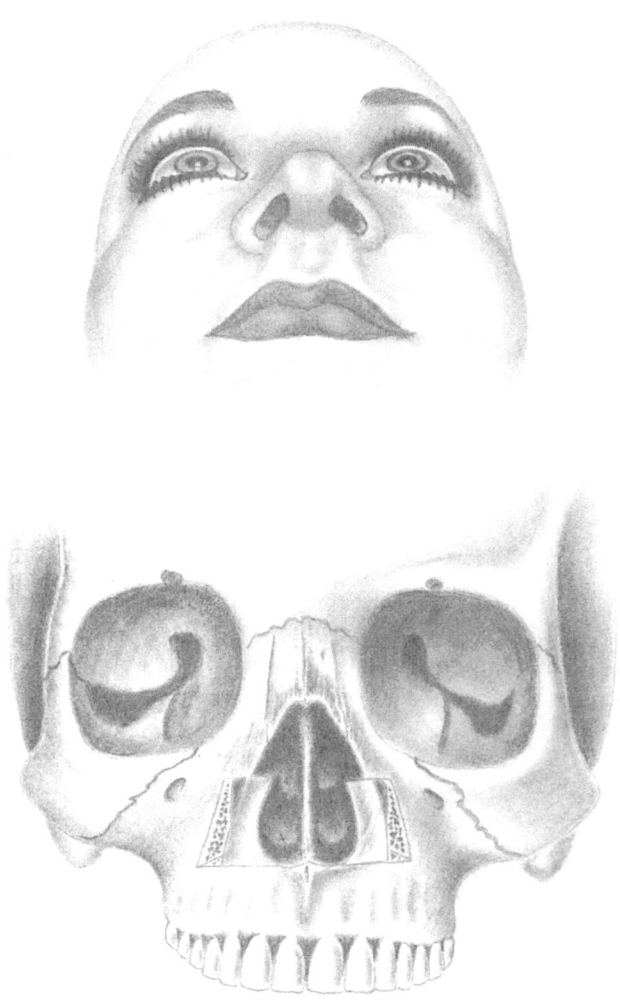

Figure 6–63

Preoperative Evaluation

The patient has retruded alae (Fig. 6-64).

Osteotomy

An upper buccal sulcus incision is used for the exposure and the periosteum is separated from the paranasal region. With an oscillating saw, the osteotomies are made as shown. The segment is pulled forward and rigid fixation is employed (Fig. 6-64).

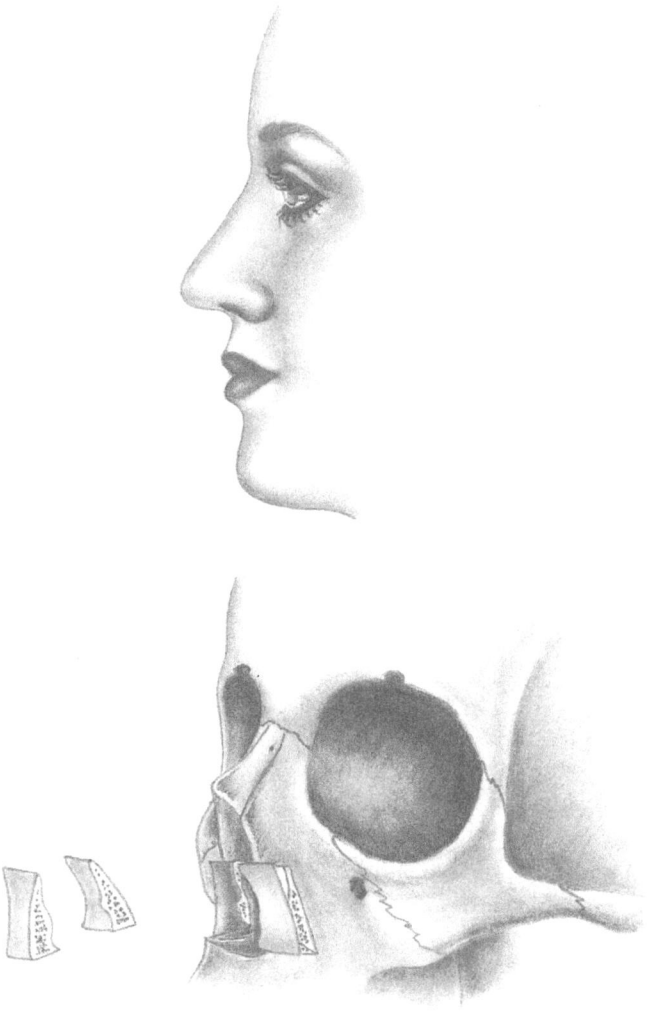

Figure 6–64

Preoperative Evaluation

On basal view, the patient has a narrow nasal base as well as narrow nares (Fig. 6-65).

Osteotomy

An upper buccal sulcus incision is made and subperiosteal dissection performed over the paranasal region. With an oscillating saw, the osteotomy at the level of the nasal floor is made. The paranasal osteotomy is performed 1 cm from the rim of the piriform aperture. Once the cuts are completed, the segment is moved laterally and rigid fixation is employed. Finally, the edge of the segment is smoothed by an oval burr (Fig. 6-65).

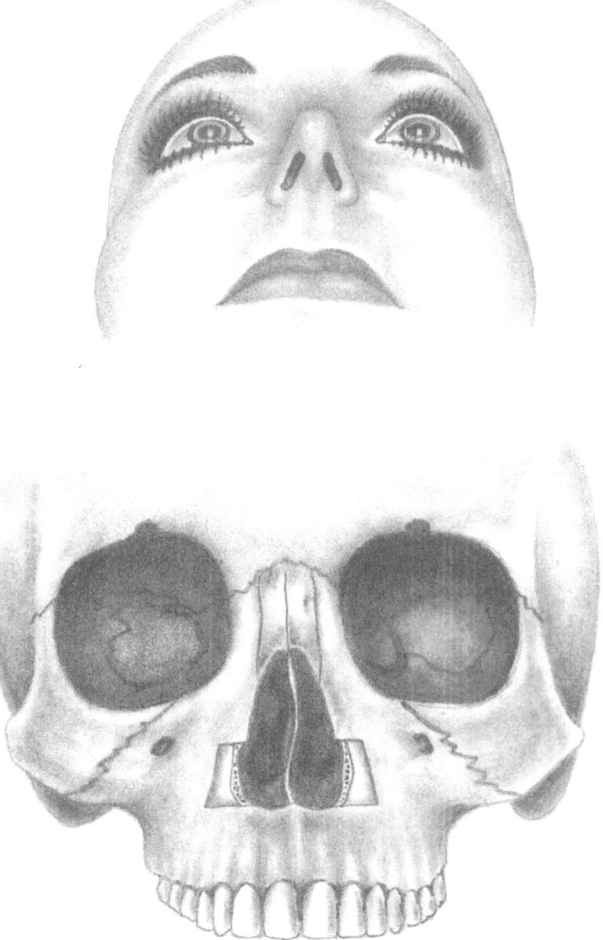

Figure 6–65

Preoperative Evaluation

On frontal view, the patient has a narrow middle vault as well as a wide nasal base. The patient also has airway impairment (Fig. 6-66).

Osteotomy

The intranasal infracartilaginous incisions are made bilaterally. The submucosal dissection is performed on the medial aspect of the bony vault and subperiosteal dissection on the paranasal region. With a curved osteotome, the paranasal osteotomy is made as shown. A greenstick fracture is made laterally on both sides (Fig. 6-66).

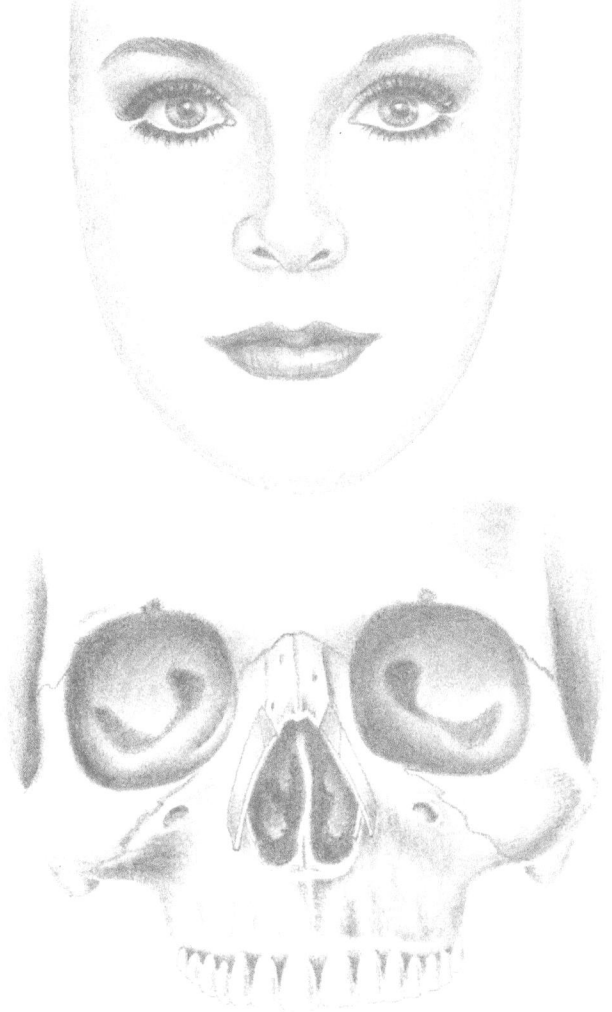

Figure 6–66

Preoperative Evaluation

The patient has a wide middle vault of the nose (Fig. 6-67).

Osteotomy

The intranasal infracartilaginous incisions are made bilaterally, and submucosal dissection is done on the medial aspect of the bony vault and subperiosteal dissection on the paranasal region. With a curved osteotome, the paranasal osteotomy is made as shown. Then the greenstick fracture is made medially from both sides (Fig. 6-67).

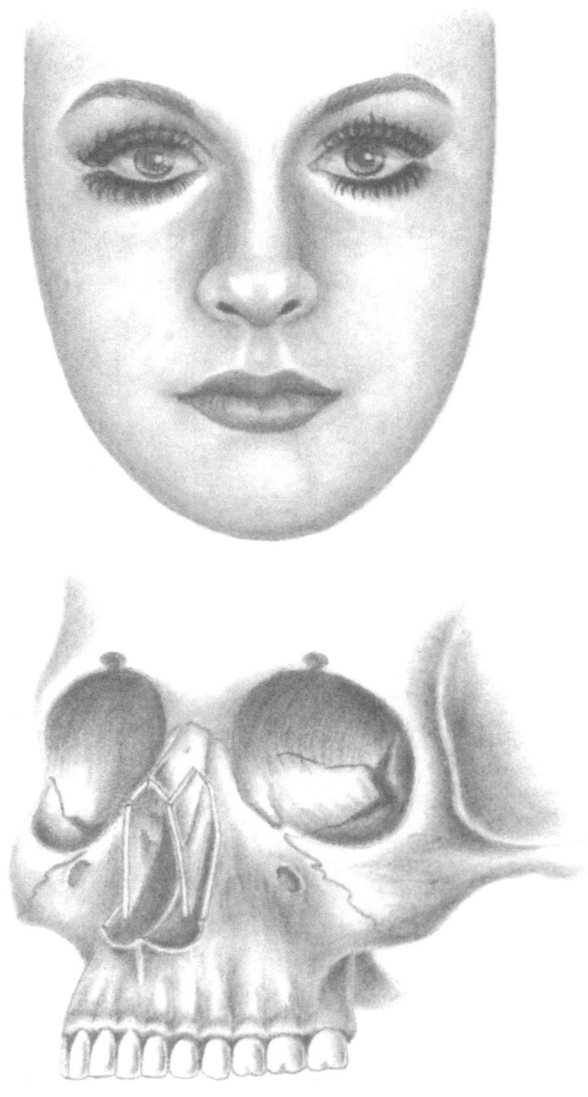

Figure 6–67

Preoperative Evaluation

On frontal view, the patient has a narrow middle vault of the nose, but the nasal airway is normal (Fig. 6-68).

Osteotomy

Initially, the bone graft is harvested and contoured. The intranasal infracartilaginous incisions are made bilaterally. The subperiosteal pocket is made at the paranasal region and the bone graft is inserted. Rigid fixation is unnecessary (Fig. 6-68).

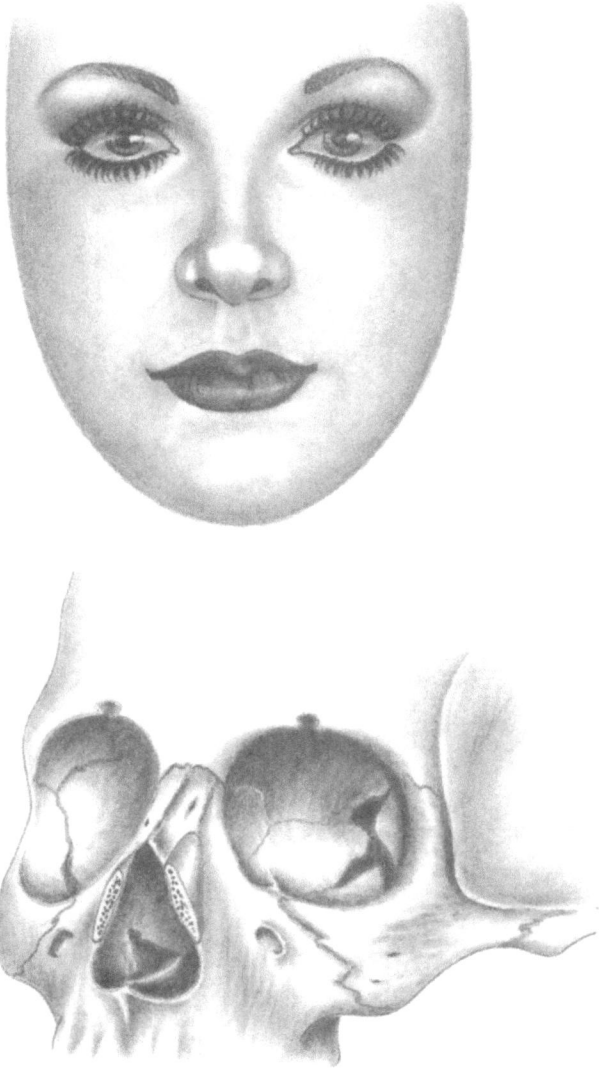

Figure 6–68

Preoperative Evaluation

On lateral view, the patient has a dorsal hump (Fig. 6-69).

Osteotomy

An intranasal infracartilaginous incision is made and subperiosteal dissection is performed over the nasal bridge. An oval burr with a guard is inserted to reduce the roof of the bony vault, which will produce an "open roof" caudal to the solid arch of bone. A fine osteotome is used to make an osteotomy as shown. The fracture is made medially to close the "open roof." Final contouring is done by a burr (Fig. 6-69).

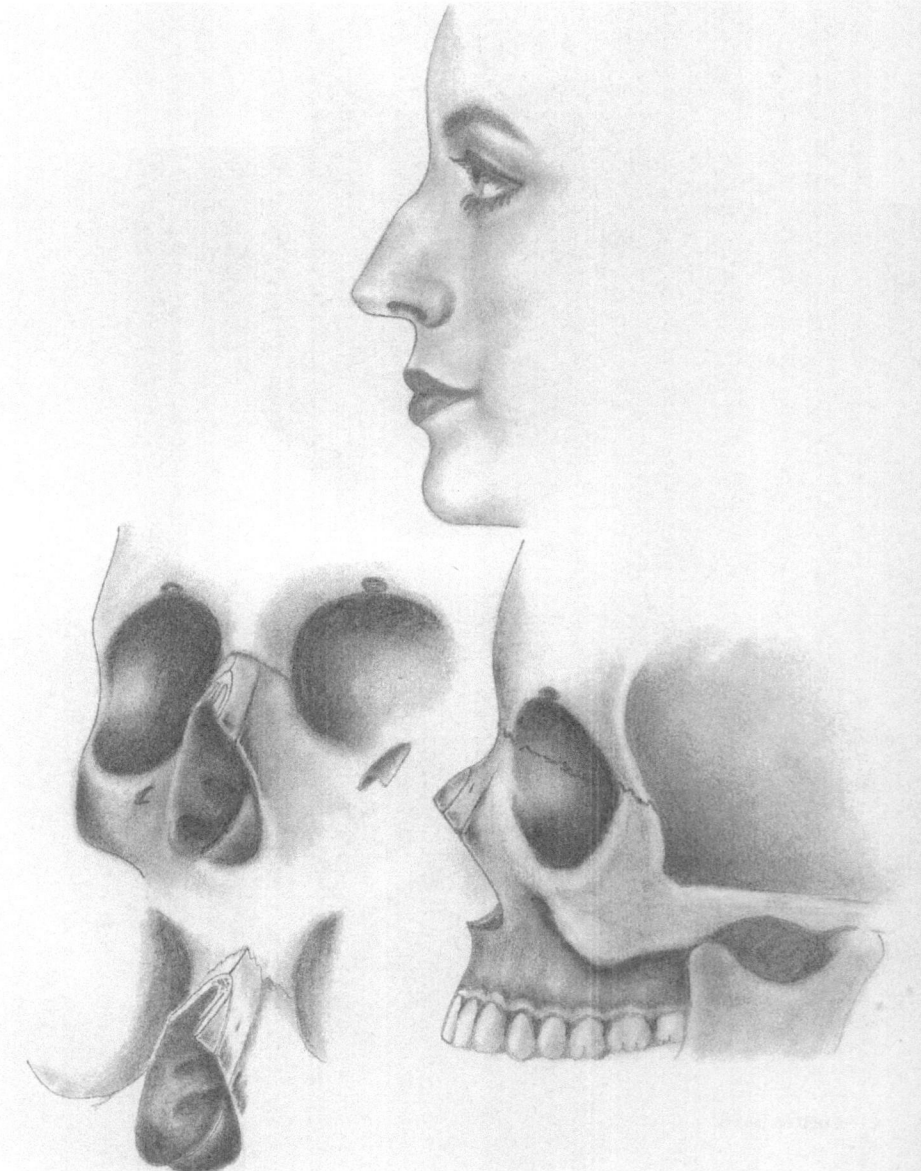

Figure 6–69

Preoperative Evaluation

On lateral view, the patient demonstrates a saddle-nose deformity (Fig. 6-70).

Osteotomy

An upper buccal sulcus incision is made and subperiosteal dissection is performed on the nasal floor, the bridge, and the paranasal regions. With a curved reciprocating saw, the paranasal osteotomy is made and a fine curved osteotome is used to transect the radix. Using a double-ball osteotome, the nasal septum is separated from the nasal floor. An elevator is inserted into the paranasal osteotomy to elevate the segment. Once the segment is moved forward, the bone graft is inserted into the gap. Rigid fixation is unnecessary (Fig. 6-70).

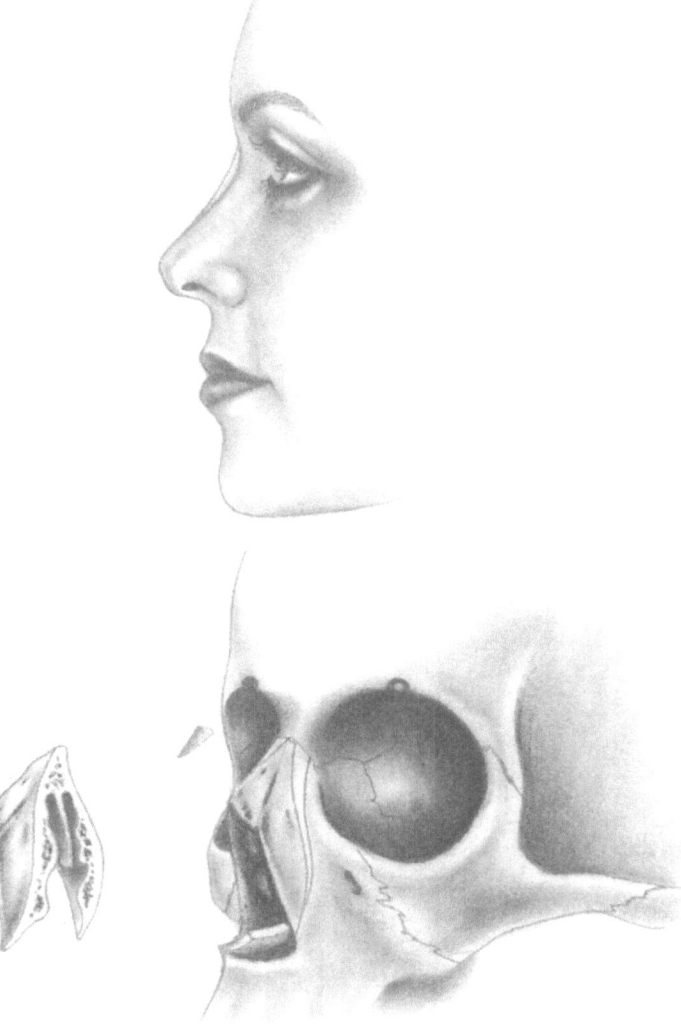

Figure 6–70

Preoperative Evaluation

This patient has a retruded nose, but the columella-labial angle is ideal (Fig. 6-71).

Osteotomy

The coronal incision is used for the exposure and subperiosteal dissection is continued to the nasal bridge, the paranasal region, and the medial orbital wall. With a right-angle oscillating saw, the paranasal osteotomies are made. With protection of the orbital contents, an osteotomy is performed on the medial orbital wall just behind the posterior lacrimal crest. The radix is transected below the level of the cribriform plate. A double-ball osteotome is inserted to separate the nasal septum from the cranial bone. Finally, the nasal septum separation at the nasal floor is made via a small vestibule incision. The segment is pulled forward and the bone graft is inserted into the gap (Fig. 6-71).

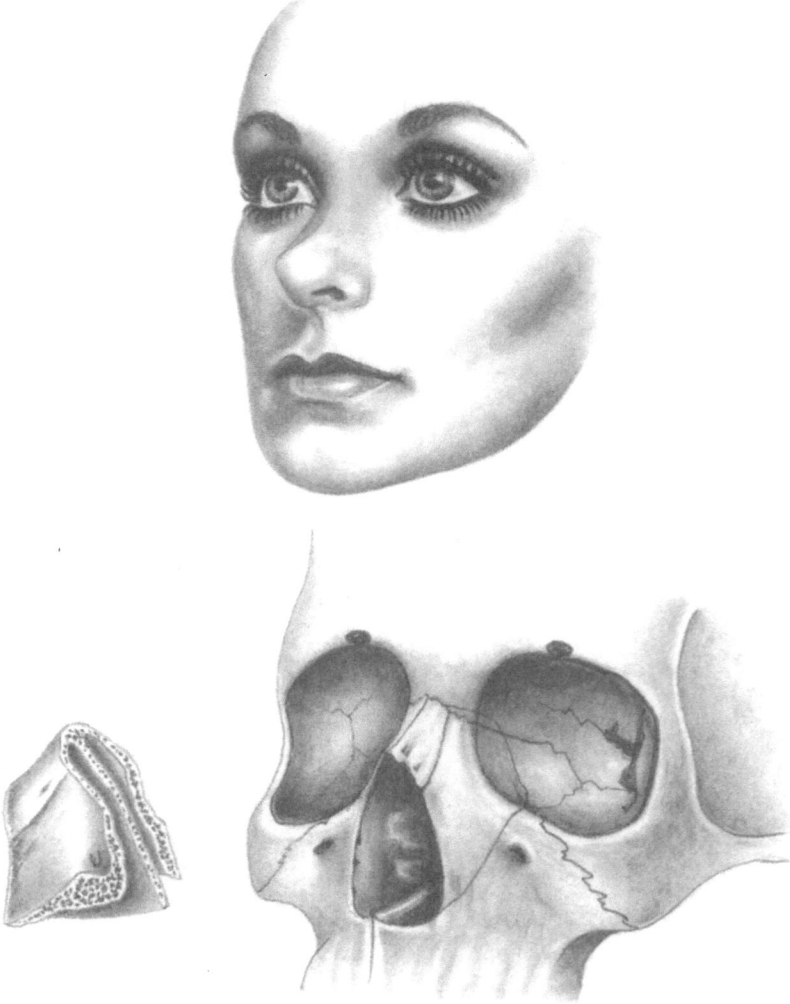

Figure 6–71

Preoperative Evaluation

The patient has a retruded nose. The columella-labial angle is less than 90° (Fig. 6-72).

Osteotomy

An upper buccal sulcus incision is made and the periosteum is separated from the subnasal region and the nasal floor. A vertical osteotomy is made on both nasal floors by a reciprocating saw. With an oscillating saw, a horizontal osteotomy is made at the subnasal region to meet the first two osteotomies on the nasal floors. Via the horizontal osteotomy, the palatal mucosa is separated from the palate. Then the coronal incision is made, and the periosteum is elevated from the nasal bridge and the paranasal region. With a reciprocating saw, the paranasal osteotomy is made. The frontonasal osteotomy is made below the level of the anterior ethmoidal foramen. The double-ball osteotome is inserted to separate the nasal septum from the cranial base. The segment is pulled forward and rigid fixation is employed (Fig. 6-72).

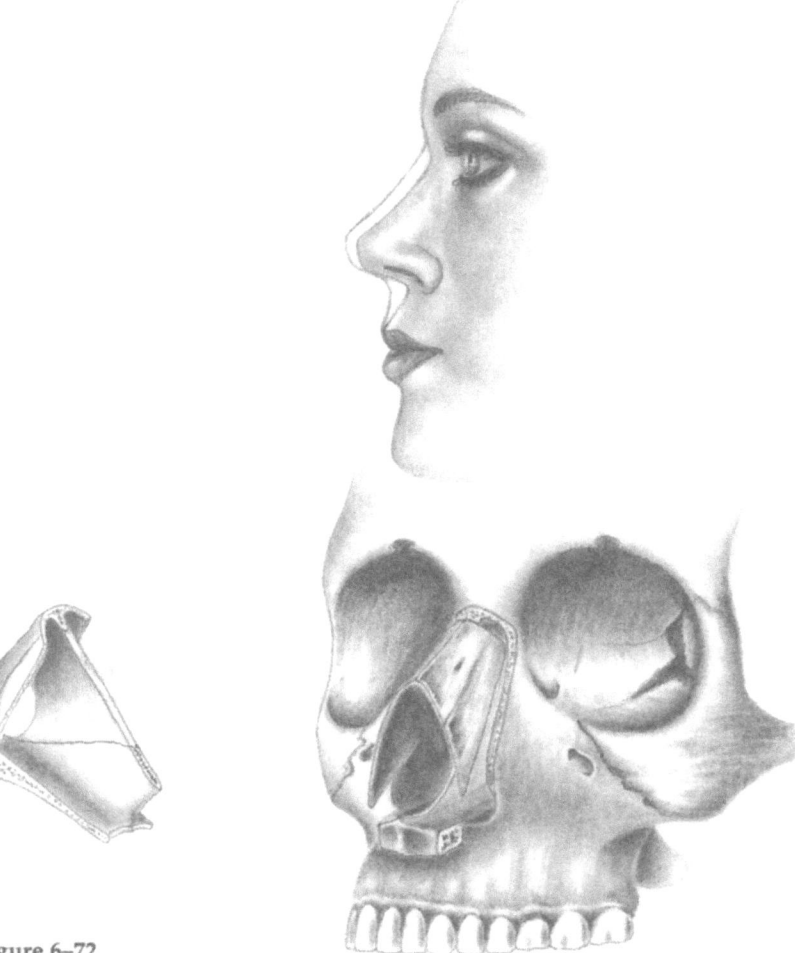

Figure 6–72

Preoperative Evaluation

The patient has a dish-like face involving the nose and the perinasal region. The occlusion is ideal (Fig. 6-73).

Osteotomy

Exposure is provided via the coronal incision and the upper buccal sulcus incision. Subperiosteal dissection is made on the nasal bridge, the nasal floor, and the subnasal and paranasal regions. With a saw-like burr, the paranasal osteotomy is performed. Then, using an oscillating saw, a horizontal osteotomy is made at the subnasal region 6 mm above the dental apices. The nasal septum is separated from the nasal floor by a double-ball osteotome. The frontonasal osteotomy is made below the level of the anterior ethmoidal foramen. The double-ball osteotome is employed to divided the nasal septum from the cranial base. Once these osteotomies are completed, the segment is pulled forward and the bone graft is inserted into the gap. Rigid fixation is employed (Fig. 6-73).

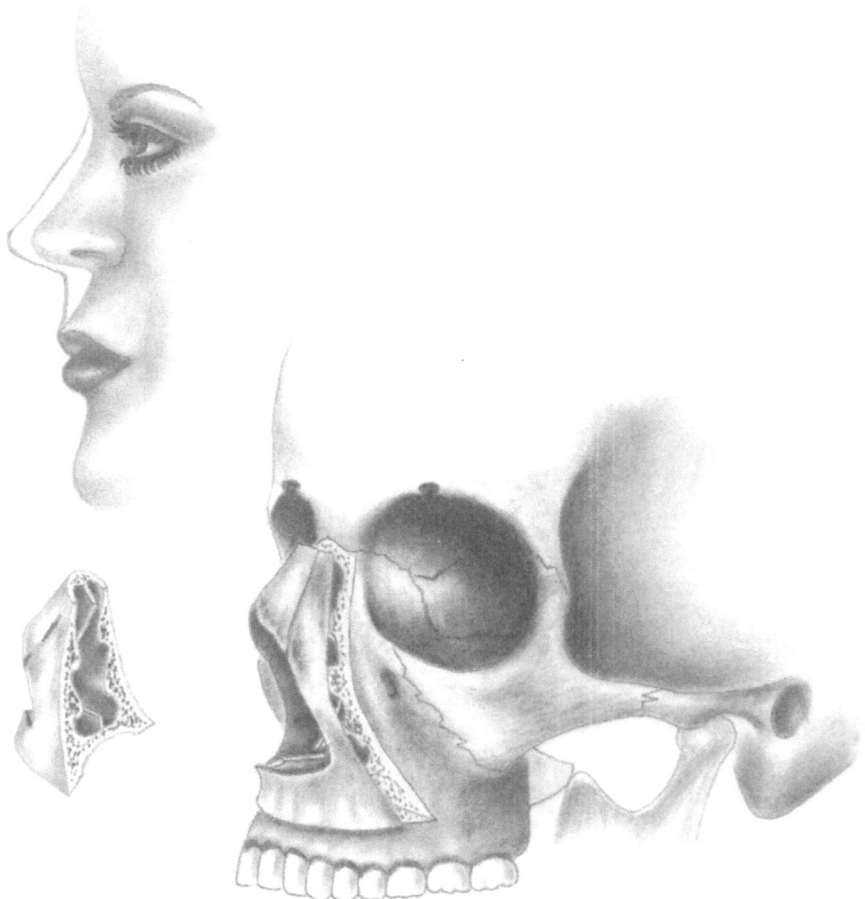

Figure 6–73

Preoperative Evaluation

The patient shows a significant deficiency at the subnasal and lateral nasal regions with a normal occlusion (Fig. 6-74).

Osteotomy

An upper buccal sulcus incision is made and subperiosteal dissection is performed on the nasal floor and the subnasal and lateral regions. With an oscillating saw, the osteotomy is made horizontally at the subnasal region 6 mm above the apices. Via this osteotomy, a fine osteotome is inserted to separate the palatal mucosa from the palate. Using a right-angle oscillating saw, the osteotomy on the paranasal region is made bilaterally. Via the paranasal osteotomy, a narrow osteotome is inserted to separate the hard palate. While the osteotomy is being performed, the surgeon's left index finger is placed against the palate from the oral cavity to palpate the osteotome tip. Penetration into the oral cavity should be avoided. With a double-ball osteotome, the nasal septum is separated from the nasal floor. The segment is pulled forward and rigid fixation is employed (Fig. 6-74).

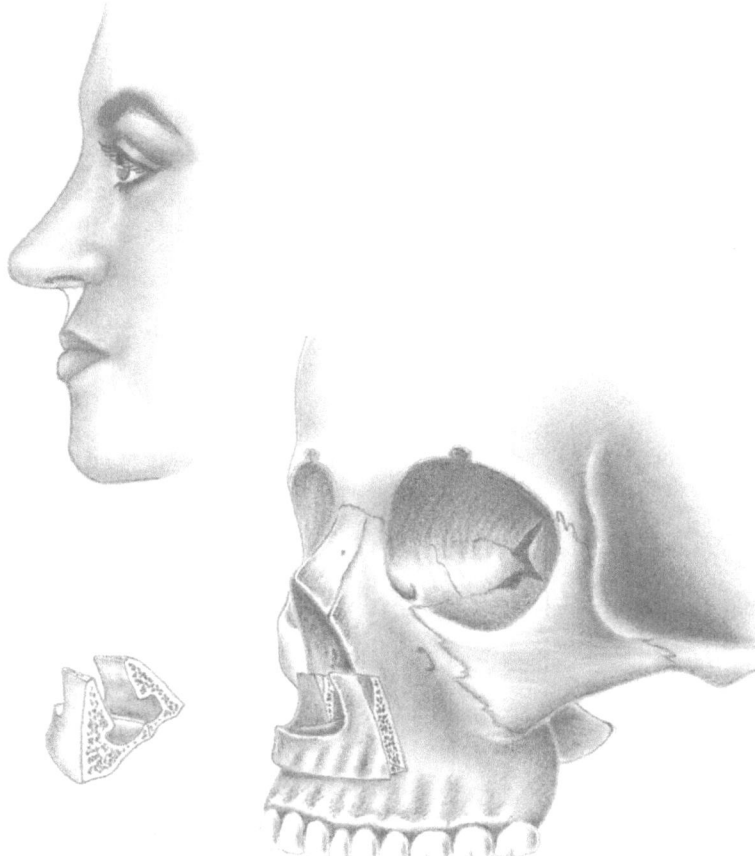

Figure 6–74

Preoperative Evaluation

This patient has a protrusion of the lower midface as well as an overjet occlusion (Fig. 6-75).

Osteotomy

The first maxillary premolar is extracted on either side. An upper buccal sulcus incision is used to expose the nasal floor and the canine fossae. With a right-angle oscillating saw, a wedge-shaped bone block is cut from the area above the extracted premolar. Using a fine osteotome, the palate is cut from either side. A double-ball osteotome is used to separate the nasal septum from the nasal floor. The segment is rotated posteriorly to obtain an ideal occlusion. Finally, rigid fixation is employed (Fig. 6-75).

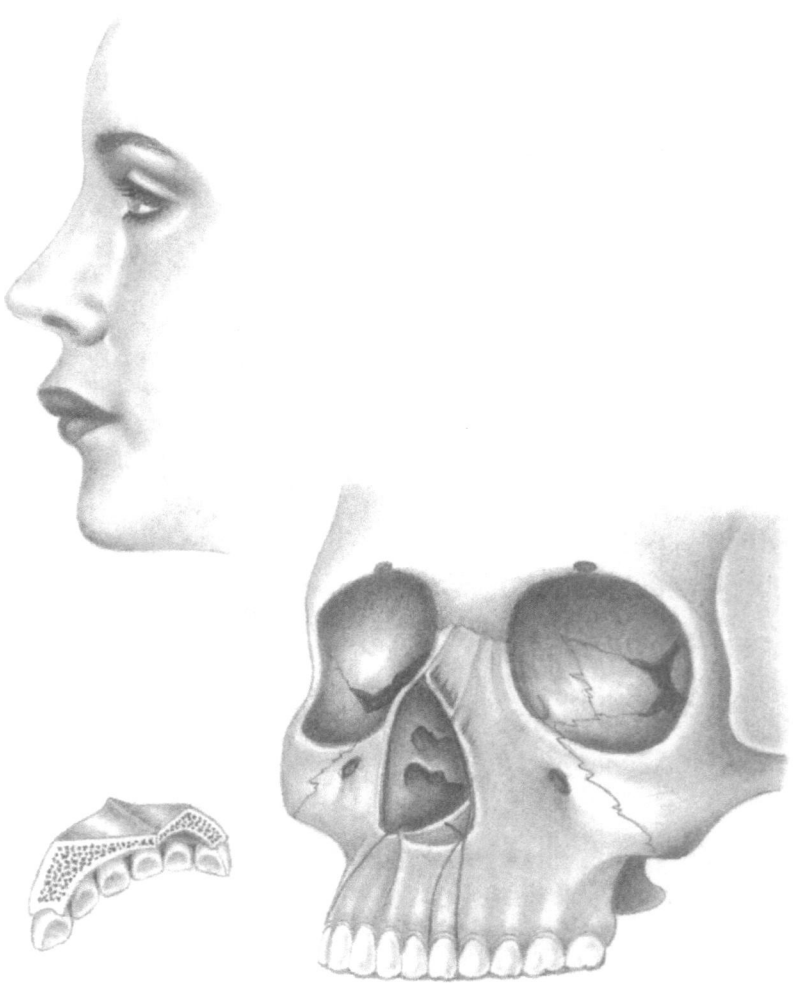

Figure 6–75

Preoperative Evaluation

The patient has a significant deficiency at the subnasal region and the canine fossae. The occlusion is ideal (Fig. 6-76).

Osteotomy

Exposure is provided via the upper buccal sulcus incision. The periosteum is elevated from the subnasal region and the nasal floor. Using an oscillating saw, a horizontal osteotomy is made at the subnasal region 6 mm above the dental apices. Via this osteotomy, the palatal mucosa is separated from the palate by a fine elevator. A narrow osteotome is used to cut the palate from either side. A double-ball osteotome is used to separate the nasal septum from the nasal floor. Once these osteotomies are completed, the segment is pulled forward to the new position. Rigid fixation is employed. An oval burr is used to smooth the frontal edge of the segment (Fig. 6-76).

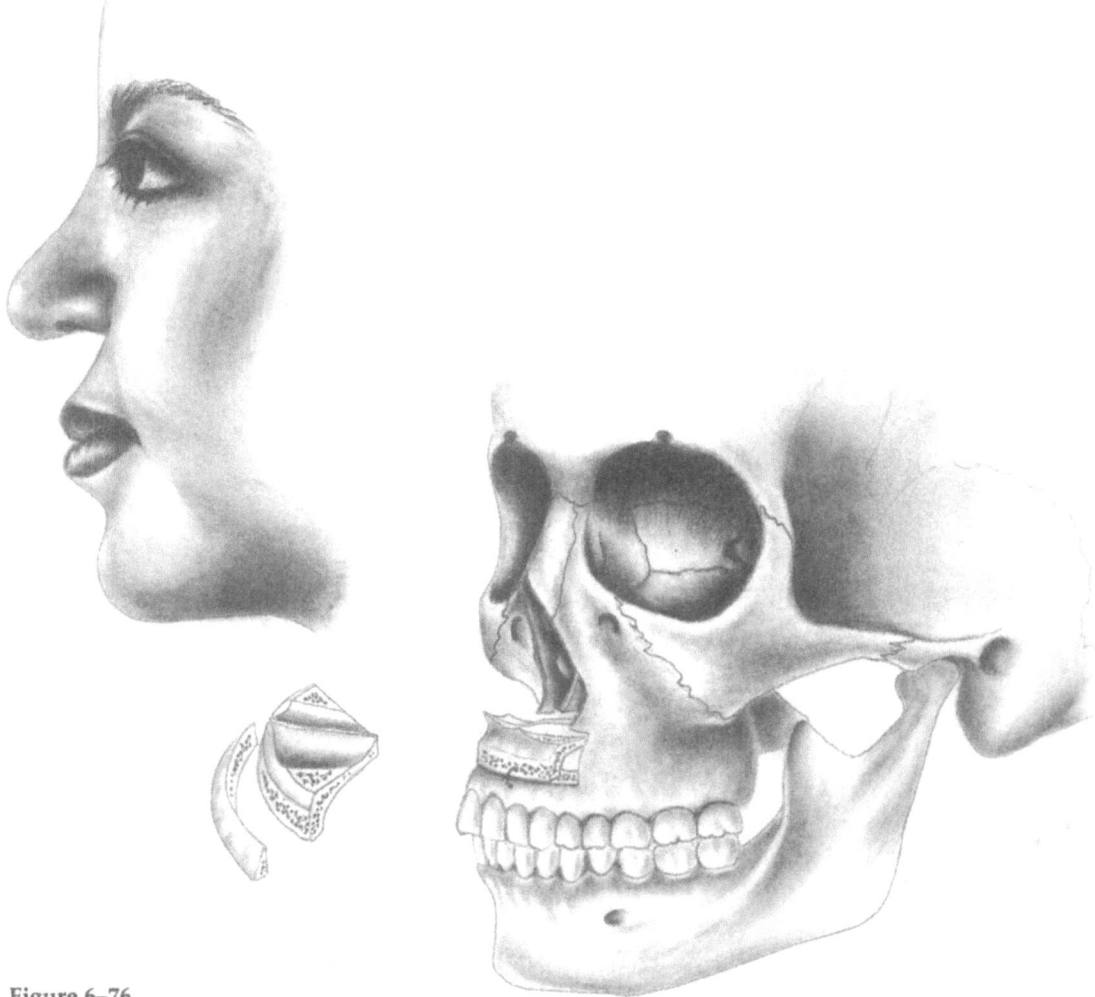

Figure 6–76

Preoperative Evaluation

The patient has a modest retrusion at the subnasal and the canine fossae, but the occlusion is normal (Fig. 6-77).

Osteotomy

The bone graft is harvested from the cranium or the rib and contoured into the predetermined shape. The upper buccal sulcus incision is made and the periosteum elevated from the subnasal region. The bone graft is inserted and screws are used for fixation. A burr is employed to smooth the bone graft edge (Fig. 6-77).

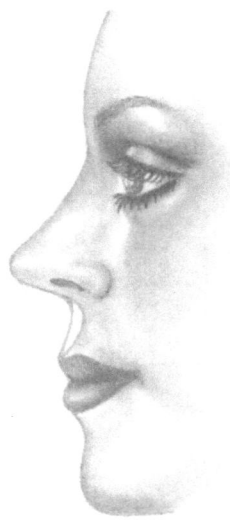

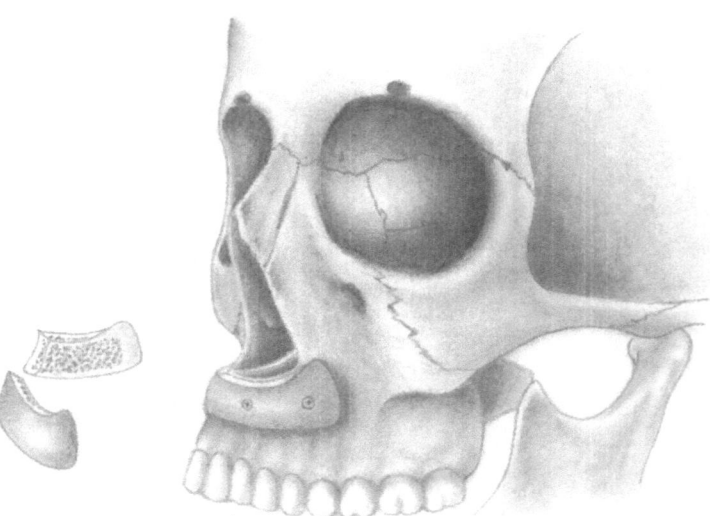

Figure 6–77

Preoperative Evaluation

On frontal view, the patient shows a narrow radix, which creates a long-nosed appearance (Fig. 6-78).

Osteotomy

The bone graft is harvested from the cranium and contoured into the desired shape. The lower blepharoplasty incision is made bilaterally. A fine curved elevator is used to dissect a pocket on the lateral radix. The bone graft is inserted and two screws are used for fixation. Asymmetry should be avoided (Fig. 6-78).

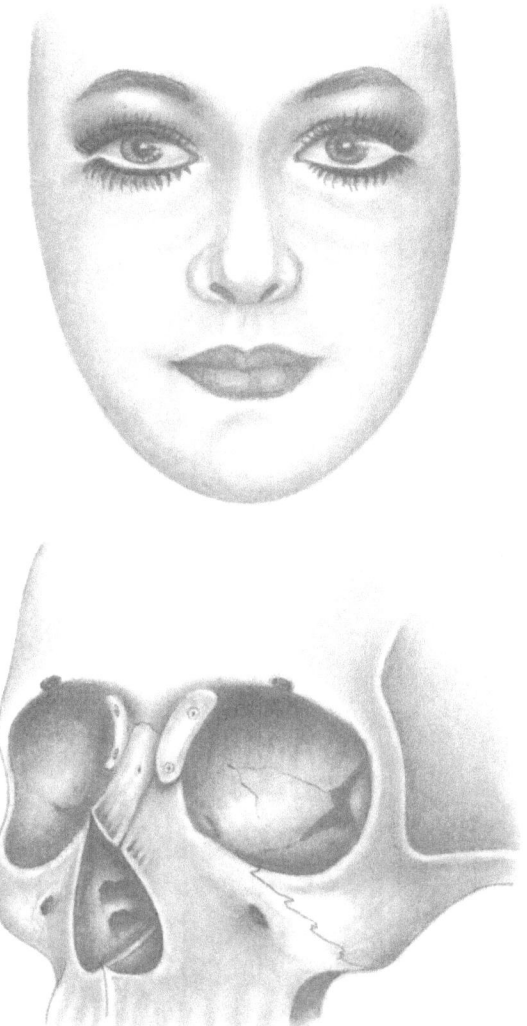

Figure 6–78

Preoperative Evaluation

On frontal view, the patient demonstrates a wide radix, which creates a short-nosed appearance (Fig. 6-79).

Osteotomy

The intranasal intercartilaginous incisions are made bilaterally. A fine elevator is inserted to separate the periosteum from the lateral radix. Then a burr with a guard is inserted to narrow the radix. Asymmetry should be avoided (Fig. 6-79).

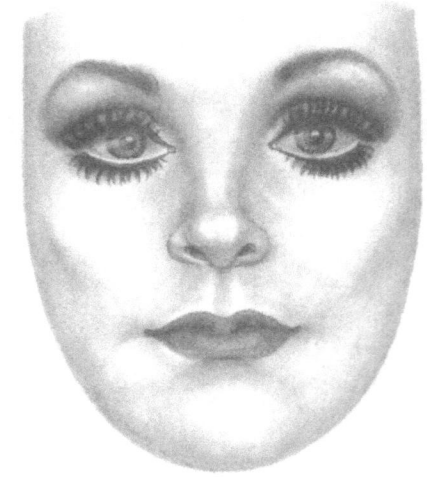

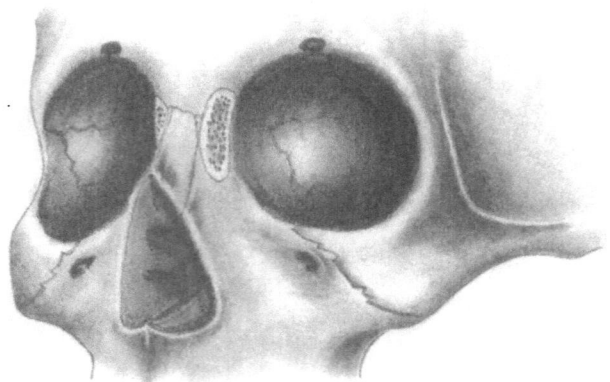

Figure 6–79

Preoperative Evaluation

On lateral view, this patient has a saddle-nose deformity (Fig. 6-80).

Osteotomy

The bone graft is harvested from the cranium and contoured. An intranasal intercartilaginous incision is made and a Penfield elevator is inserted to separate the periosteum from the bridge and the radix. Care must be taken to create a pocket the proper size for the bone graft. A too-large pocket will allow for graft movement. The bone graft is inserted. Fixation is unnecessary (Fig. 6-80).

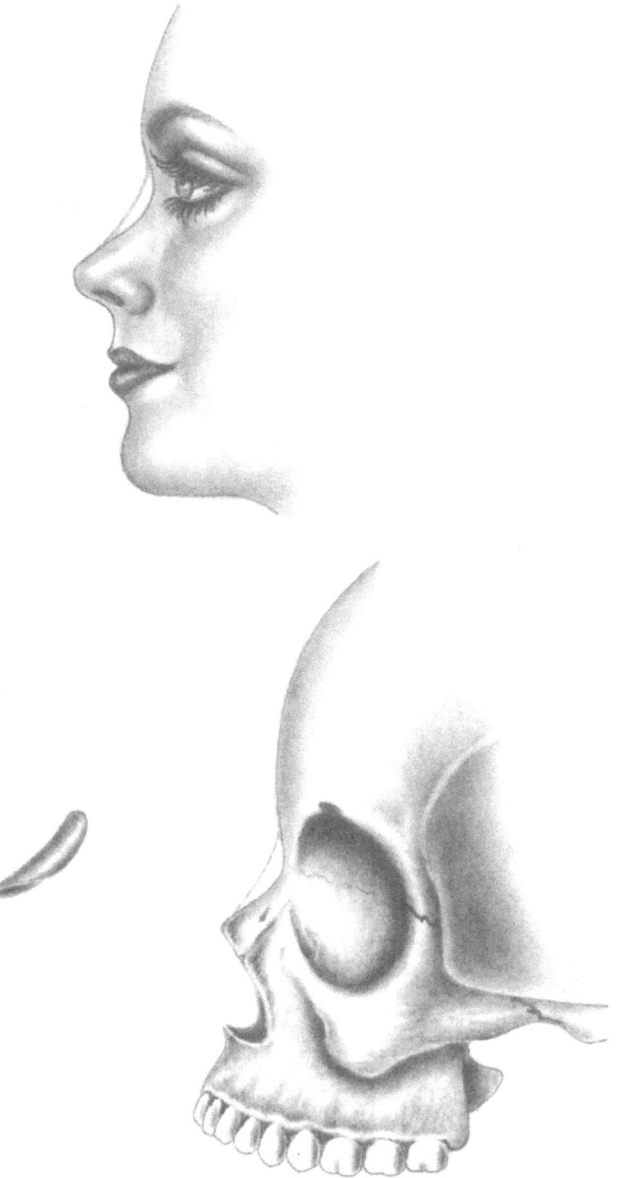

Figure 6–80

Preoperative Evaluation

On lateral view, the patient demonstrates a high nasal radix (Fig. 6-81).

Osteotomy

An intranasal intercartilaginous incision is made and a Penfield elevator is inserted to separate the periosteum from the bridge and the radix. An oval burr with a guard is used to reduce the radix. Overcorrection should be avoided (Fig. 6-81).

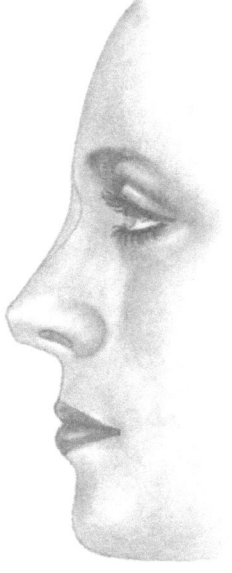

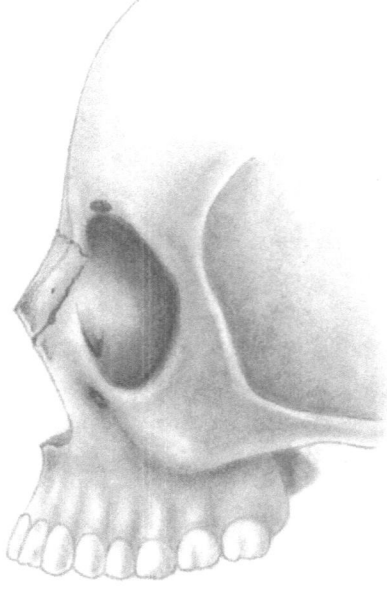

Figure 6–81

Malar Region

Preoperative Evaluation

The patient has exophthalmos with underdeveloped malar eminences (Fig. 6-82).

Osteotomy

Exposure is provided via the coronal incision with subperiosteal dissection to the lateral orbital rims and the zygomatic arches and buttress. With the orbital contents protected, the lateral orbital wall and the zygomatic arch are cut by a reciprocating saw via the temporal fossa. Using a right-angle oscillating saw, the osteotomies on the paranasal regions and the zygomatic buttress are made. Once these cuts are completed, the segment is pulled forward and rigid fixation is employed along the anterior osteotomy lines (Fig. 6-82).

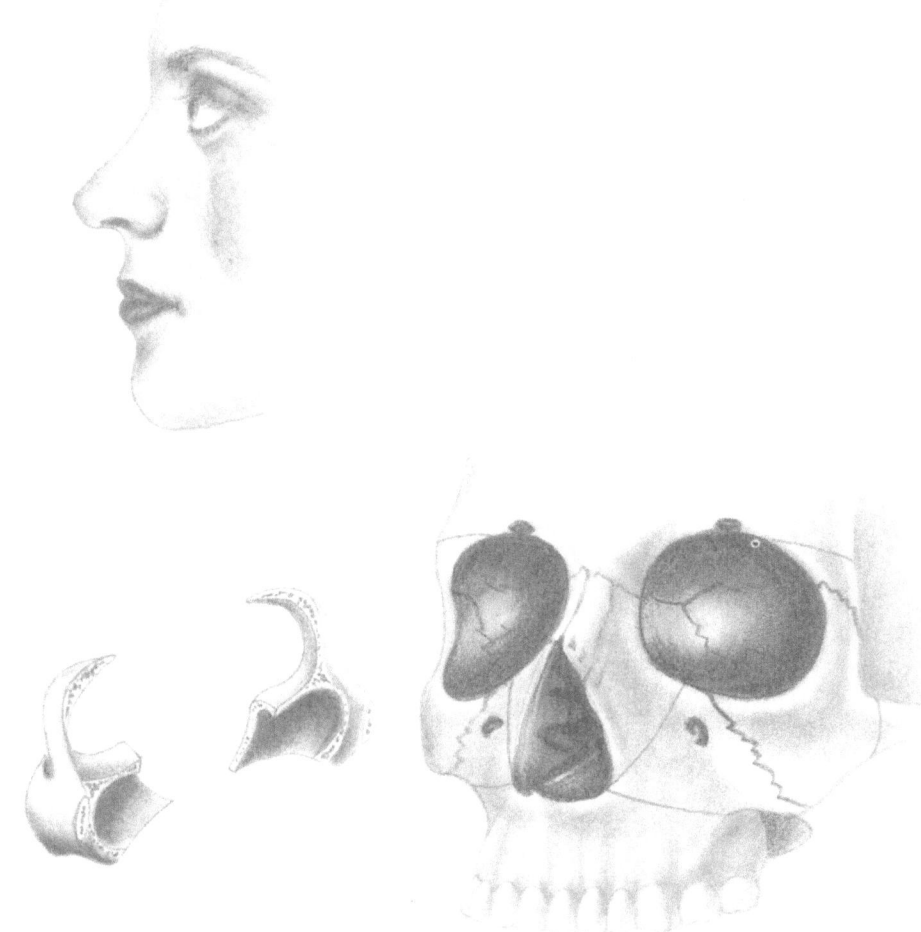

Figure 6–82

Preoperative Evaluation

This patient shows a lateral protrusion of the zygoma and the arches (Fig. 6-83).

Osteotomy

The upper buccal sulcus incision is made and the periosteum is elevated from the anterior-lateral surface of the zygoma. The volume that is to be reduced from the lateral zygoma is determined and marked. With a reciprocating saw, a wedge-shaped osteotomy that is wider superiorly than inferiorly and wider anteriorly than posteriorly is cut from the lateral zygomatic region bilaterally. Via a preauricular stab wound, a greenstick fracture is made on the zygomatic arch posteriorly to where it starts protruding laterally, and the segment is moved medially. Wires are used at the anterior rim for fixation (Fig. 6-83).

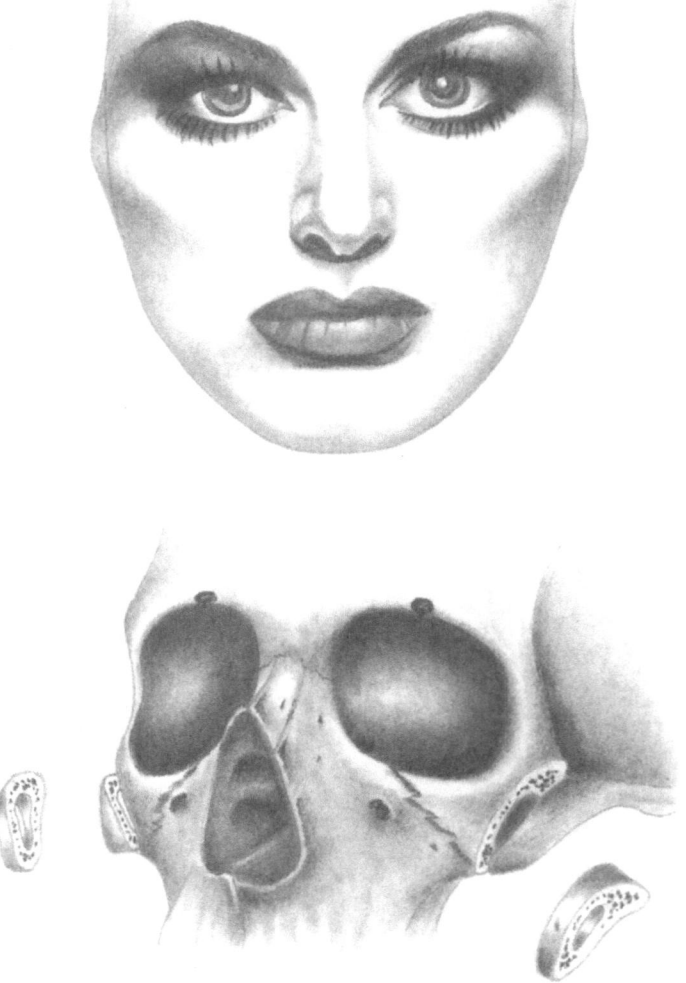

Figure 6–83

Preoperative Evaluation

The patient presents a lateral protrusion of the zygoma (Fig. 6-84).

Osteotomy

The upper buccal sulcus incision is made bilaterally. Subperiosteal dissection is performed on the lateral surface of the zygoma, posterior to the zygomatic arch where the masseter muscle attaches. With an oscillating saw, the lateral portion of the zygoma is sagittally cut at the desired position. The window of the maxillary sinus is checked. A proper bone graft is selected from the segment and replaced over the window. Wire is used at the anterior rim for fixation (Fig. 6-84).

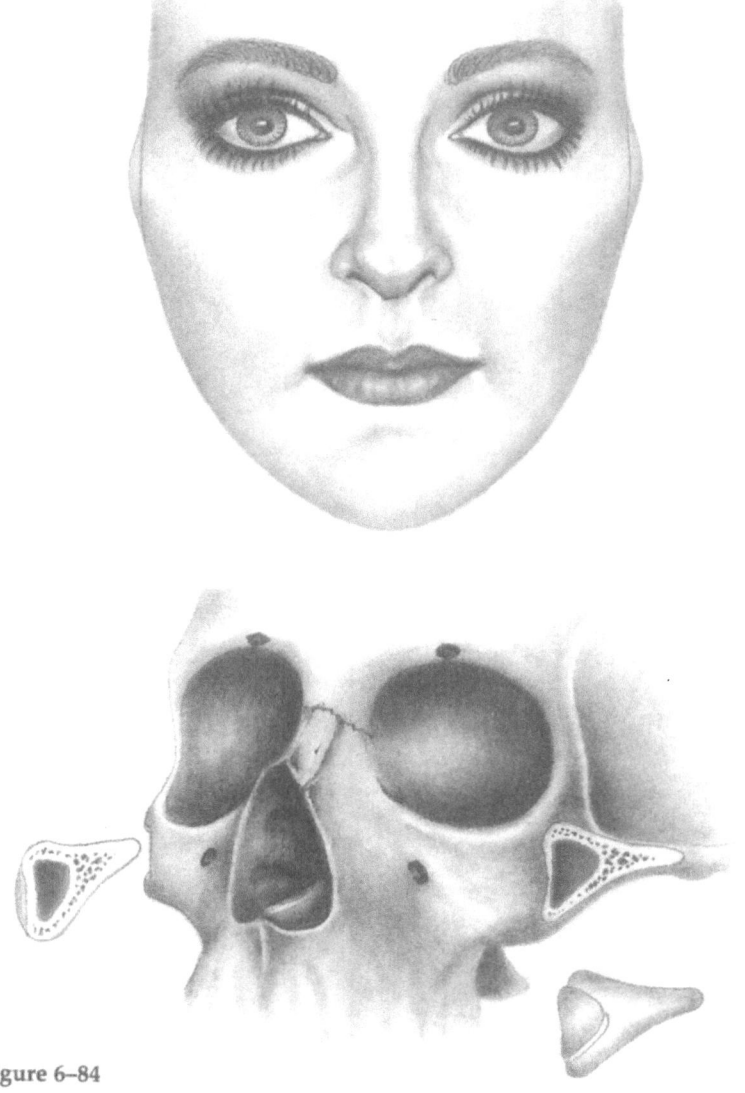

Figure 6–84

Preoperative Evaluation

The patient shows an anterior deficiency of the zygoma (Fig. 6-85).

Osteotomy

The upper buccal sulcus incision is made. With a reciprocating saw, the anterior wall of the maxillary sinus is cut along the coronal plane. Care must be taken to prevent injuring the infraorbital nerve. An osteotome with a wide edge is inserted into the gap to elevate the segment and the predetermined bone graft is placed in the gap. Wires are used at the inferior rim for fixation (Fig. 6-85).

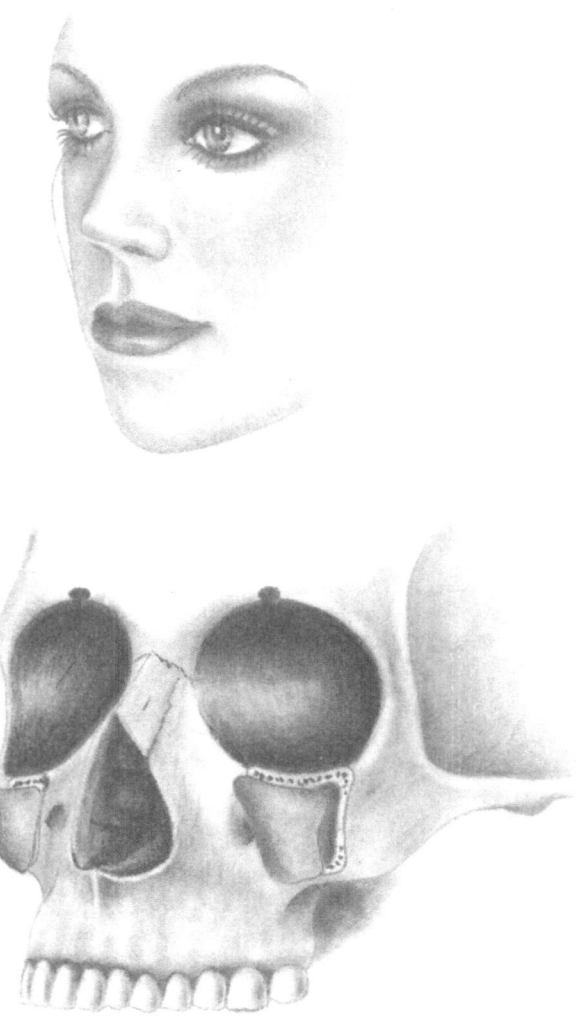

Figure 6–85

Preoperative Evaluation

The patient has a relative anterior-lateral protrusion of the zygoma (Fig. 6-86).

Osteotomy

The upper buccal sulcus incision is made and the periosteum is elevated from the zygomatic surface. With a reciprocating saw, the protruded portion of the zygoma is cut as shown. The window of the maxillary sinus is identified and a proper bone graft is selected from the removed segment and replaced over the window. Wires are used for fixation (Fig. 6-86).

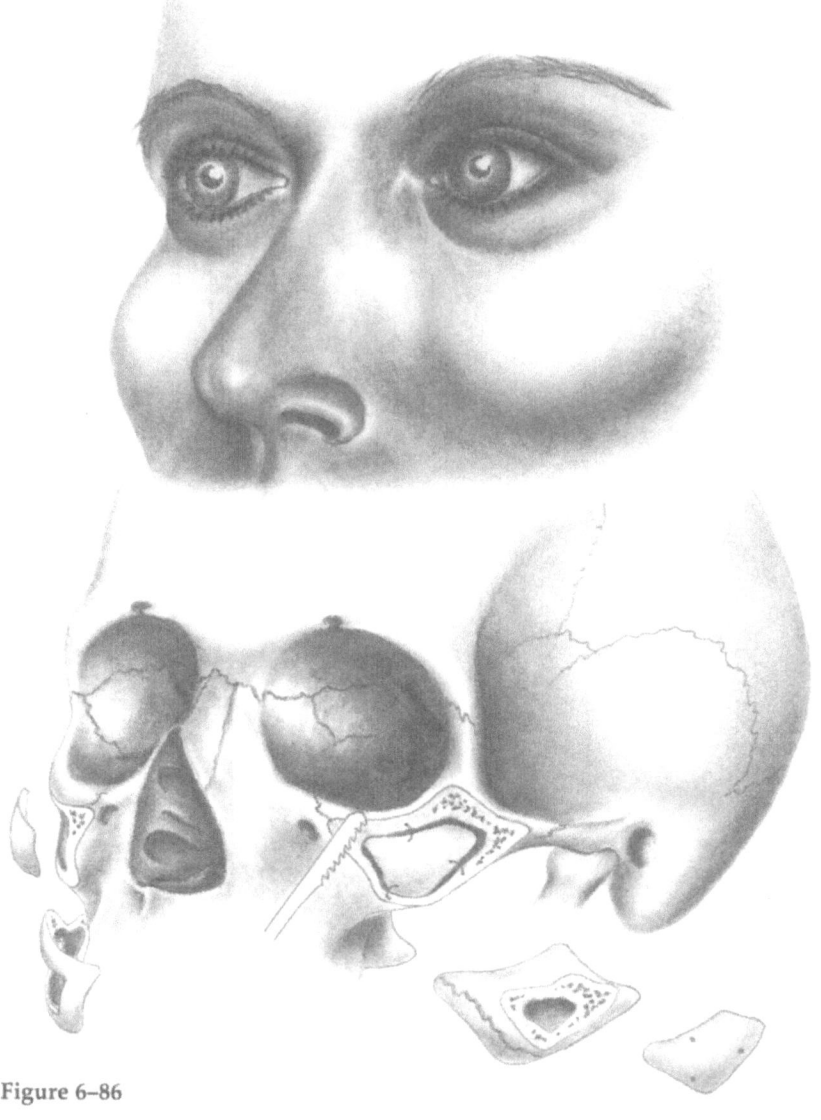

Figure 6–86

Preoperative Evaluation

On frontal view, the patient shows a deficiency of the midfacial width. The malar eminences are well-developed in the anterior direction (Fig. 6-87).

Osteotomy

The exposure is provided via the upper buccal sulcus incision. With an oscillating saw, the lateral portion of the zygoma is cut vertically as shown. A wider osteotome is inserted into the gap to elevate the segment laterally. A greenstick fracture is made at the posterior portion of the segment and the bone graft with the desired width is placed in the gap. Fixation is unnecessary (Fig. 6-87).

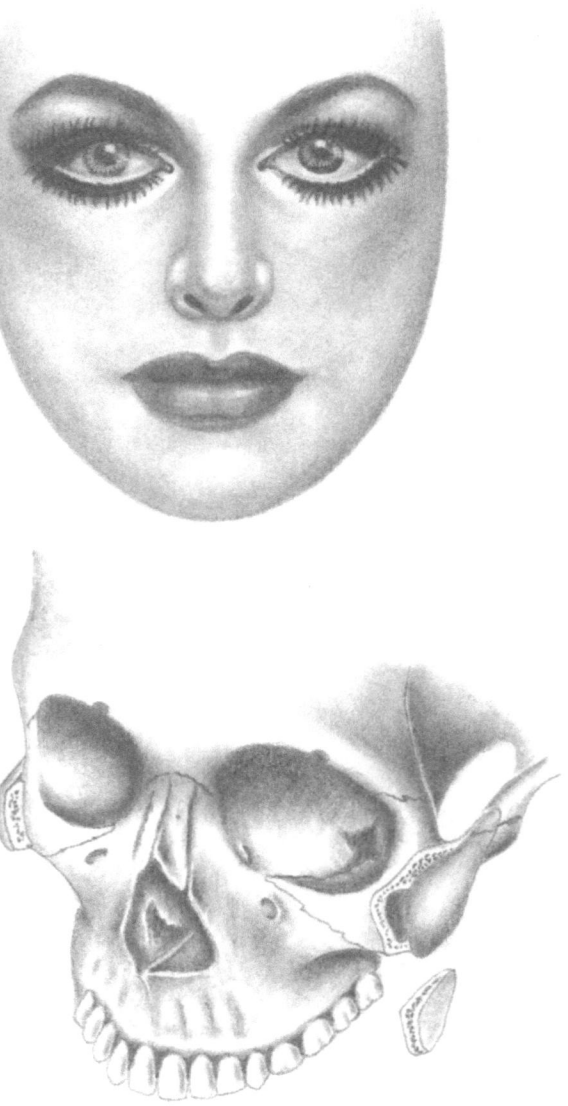

Figure 6–87

Preoperative Evaluation

On oblique view, the patient has a flat cheek with a retrusion of the infraorbital rim (Fig. 6-88).

Osteotomy

The lower blepharoplasty incision is made for the exposure. Subperiosteal dissection is carried out over the orbital floor and the zygomatic surface and arch. With the orbital contents protected, the orbital floor and the lateral orbital rim are cut by a right-angle oscillating saw with a short blade. A fine curved osteotome is used to cut the lateral wall of the maxillary sinus via the same incision. With a reciprocating saw through an upper buccal sulcus incision, the lateral to the infraorbital foramen osteotomy is performed vertically on the anterior maxillary sinus wall to meet the osteotomy on the orbital floor. Finally, the zygomatic arch is cut. The segment is pulled forward and rigid fixation is employed (Fig. 6-88).

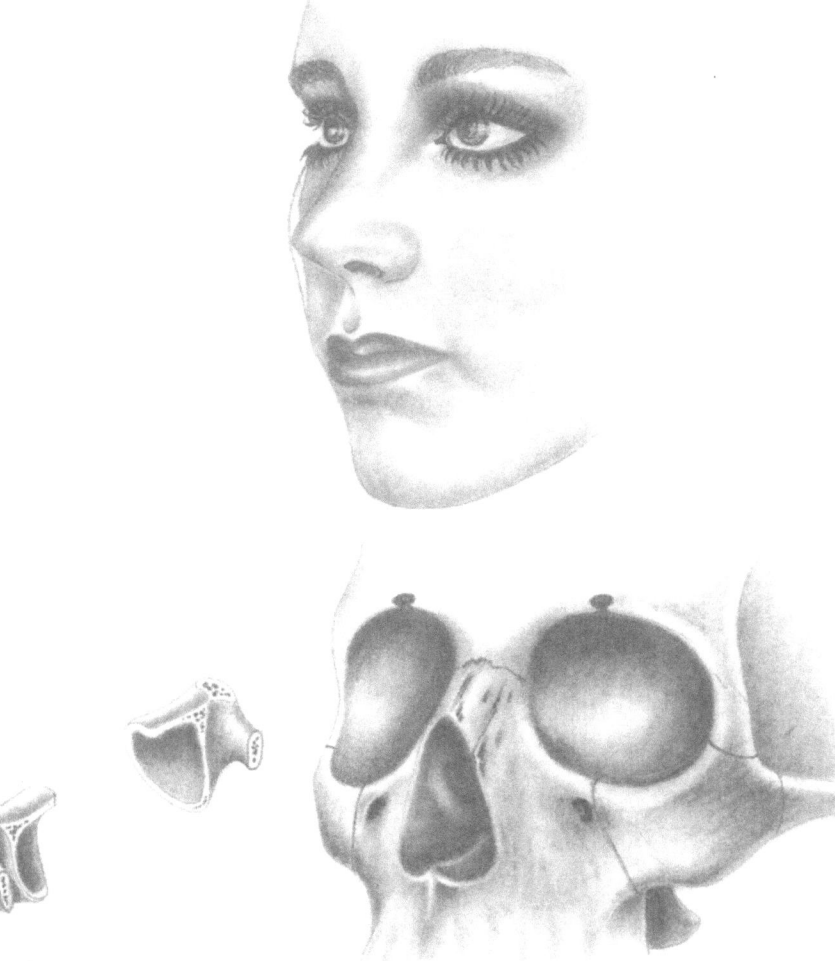

Figure 6–88

Preoperative Evaluation

On oblique view, the patient presents a flat cheek and depression at the submalar area (Fig. 6-89).

Osteotomy

The upper buccal sulcus incision is made bilaterally and subperiosteal dissection is performed over the malar surface, posteriorly to the zygomatic arch where the masseter muscle attaches. With a reciprocating saw, the osteotomy is performed on the malar eminence, across the frontal portion of the maxillary sinus, entering the temporal fossa. The zygomatic arch is cut as shown. The segment is moved anterior-inferiorly. Miniplates are used for fixation. A small burr is used to smooth the edge of the segment (Fig. 6-89).

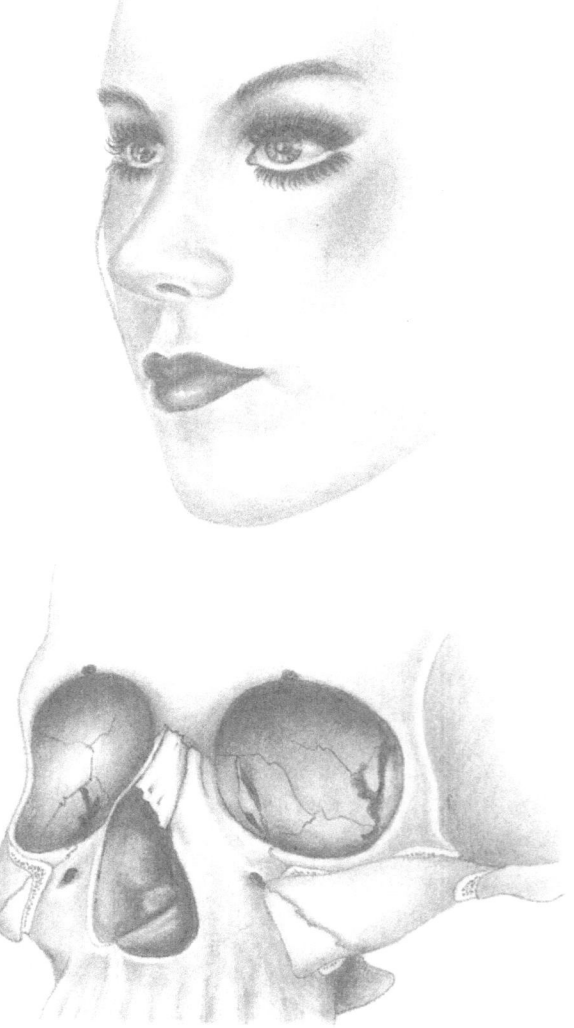

Figure 6–89

Preoperative Evaluation

The patient has a depression at the anterior submalar area (Fig. 6-90).

Osteotomy

The cranial bone graft is harvested and contoured. A small upper buccal sulcus incision is made bilaterally. Subperiosteal dissection is carried out over the anterior-inferior surface of the zygoma. The bone graft is placed over the canine fossa and adjusted in the desired position. Two screws are used for fixation. Frequently, an oval burr is needed to trim and smooth the edge of the bone graft (Fig. 6-90).

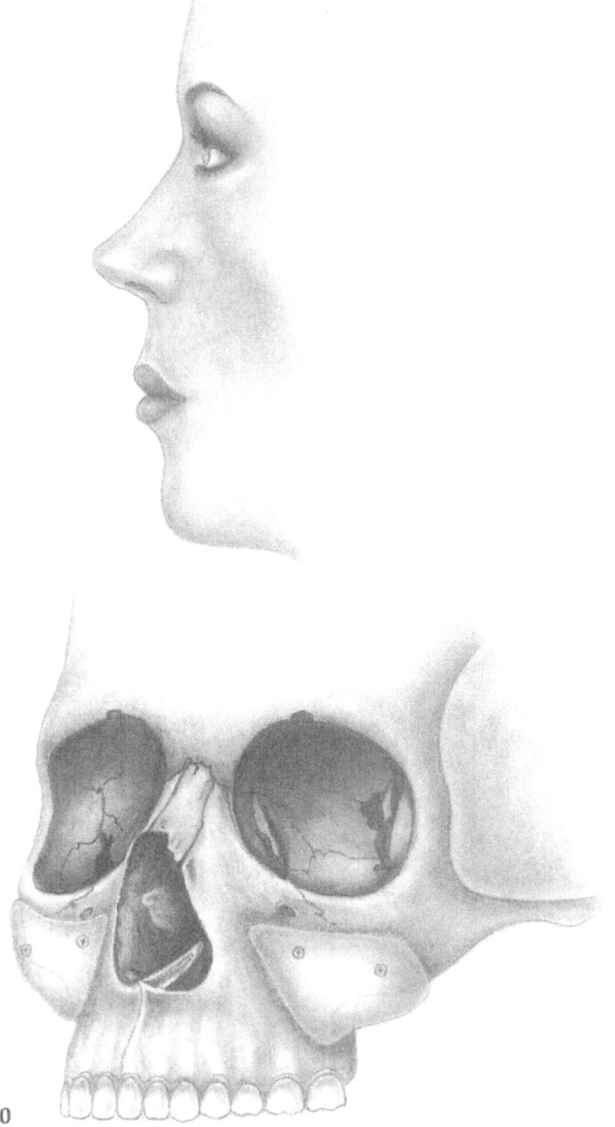

Figure 6–90

Preoperative Evaluation

The patient shows a gaunt appearance with marked hollows and depressions at the submalar areas (Fig. 6-91).

Osteotomy

Firstly, the cranial bone graft is harvested and contoured to the predetermined shape. A small incision is made at the upper buccal sulcus bilaterally, and subperiosteal dissection is performed over the lateral malar surface. The bone graft is inserted into the pocket and two screws are used for fixation. Asymmetry should be avoided (Fig. 6-91).

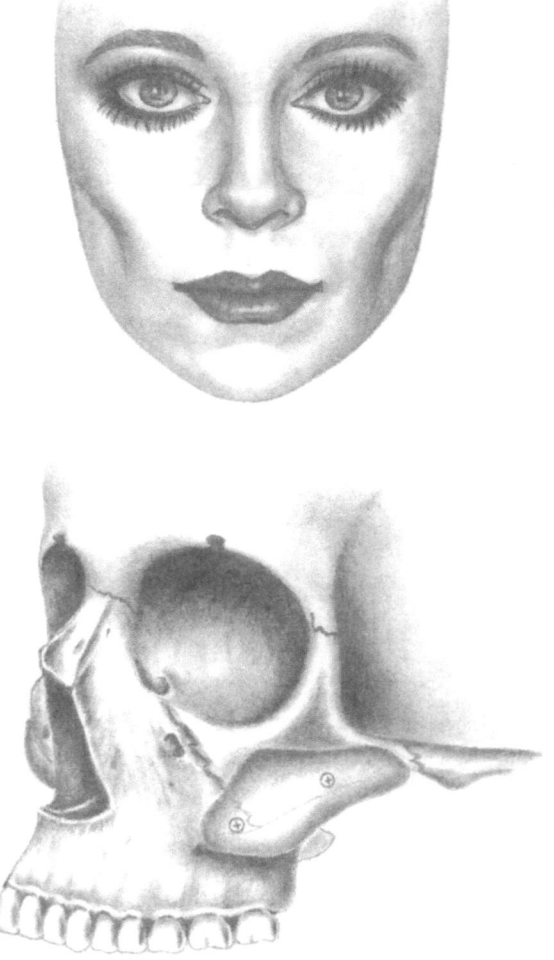

Figure 6–91

Preoperative Evaluation

The patient has deep nasolabial folds and a depression at the anterior maxillary area (Fig. 6-92).

Osteotomy

The cranial bone graft is harvested and contoured. The upper buccal sulcus incision is made bilaterally and the periosteum is elevated from the canine fossa. The bone graft is inserted into the pocket and several screws are employed for fixation (Fig. 6-92).

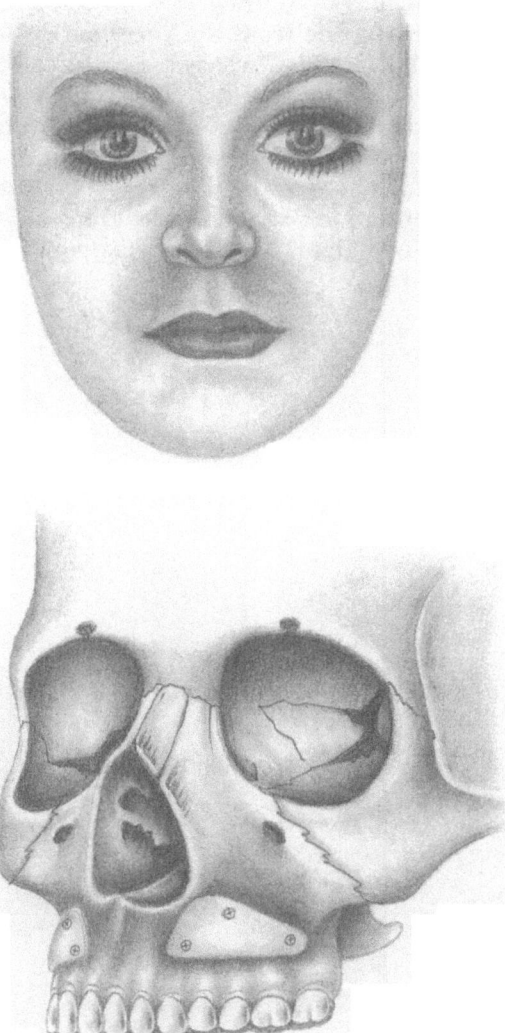

Figure 6–92

Maxillary Region

Preoperative Evaluation

The patient shows a vertical shortness of the lower midface. The incisors do not show while smiling (Fig. 6-93).

Osteotomy

An upper buccal sulcus incision is made from the first molar region on one side to the equal position on the opposite. The periosteum is elevated off the maxilla at the level of the piriform aperture. The nasal mucosa is separated from the floor of the nose and the vomerine groove. With a small reciprocating saw, an osteotomy is made transversely across the maxilla from the pterygomaxillary fissure to the piriform margin bilaterally. The nasal septum is separated from the vomerine groove by a double-ball osteotome, and using a curved osteotome, the pterygoid plate and maxillary tuberosity are separated. A down-fracture is made and the maxilla is completely mobilized. The cranial, rib, or iliac bone graft can be inserted into the gap for lengthening and rigid fixation is preferred to decrease resorption or change in vertical height of the bone (Fig. 6-93).

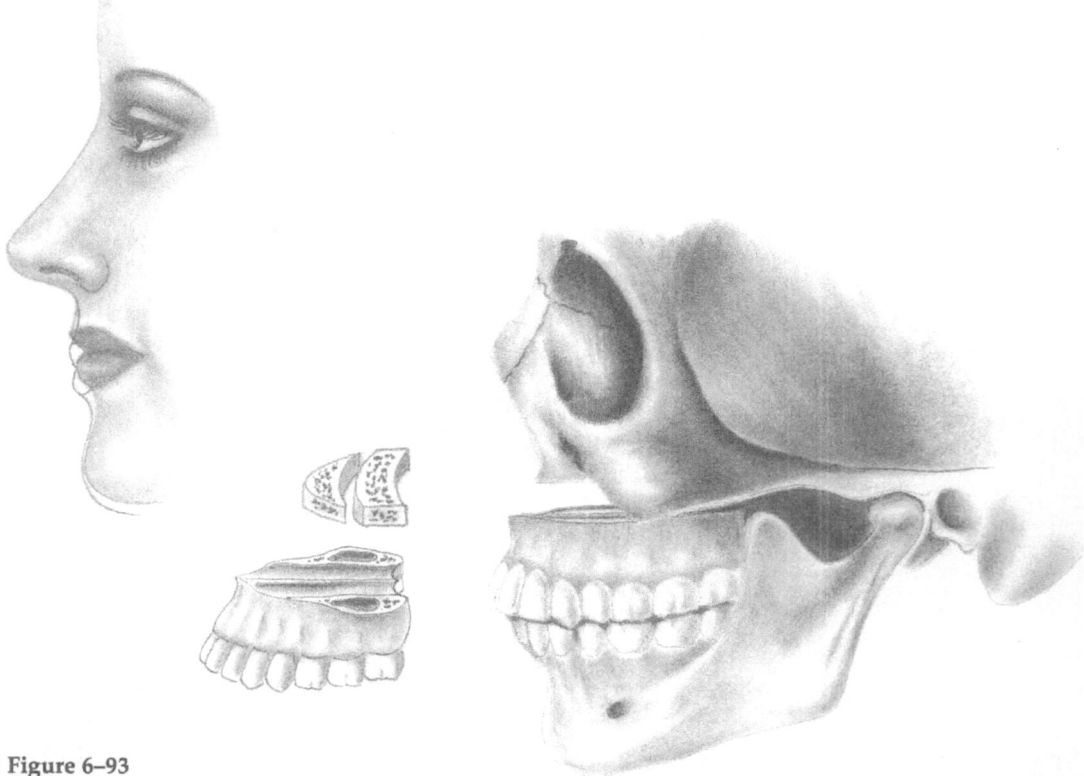

Figure 6–93

Preoperative Evaluation

This patient has a retrusion of the lower midface with a class III occlusion (Fig. 6-94).

Osteotomy

A lower Le Fort I osteotomy is used for the treatment of this deformity with the approach in the upper buccal sulcus. The subperiosteal dissection is made below the anterior nasal spine. An oscillating saw is used to cut horizontally the maxilla at least 6 mm above the dental apices. With a curved osteotome, the junction of the tuberosity and pterygoid plates are separated and the segment is advanced to obtain an ideal occlusion and a well-balanced face (Fig. 6-94).

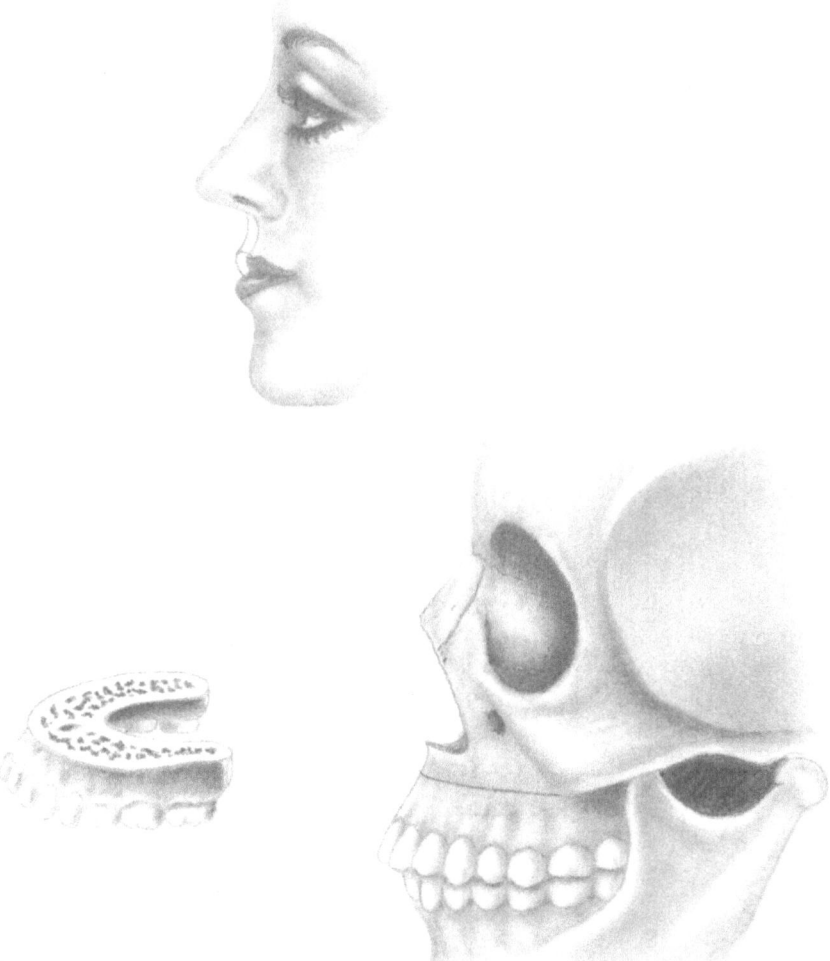

Figure 6–94

Preoperative Evaluation

This patient has a long and retruded lower midface as well as a class III occlusion deformity (Fig. 6-95).

Osteotomy

A variation of a Le Fort I osteotomy (from a high anterior to a low posterior position) is used for the treatment of this deformity. Except for the osteotomy direction, the procedure is the same as the low Le Fort I osteotomy. This osteotomy shortens the maxilla as it is moved forward (Fig. 6-95).

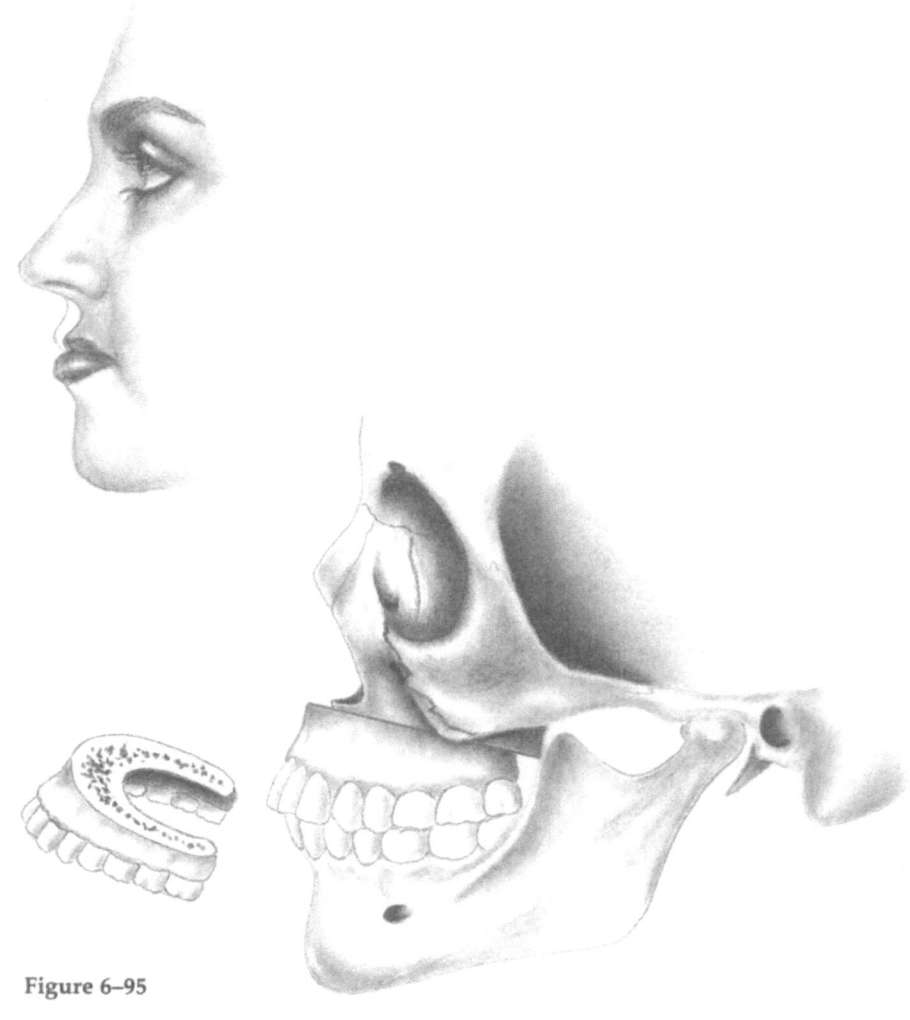

Figure 6–95

Preoperative Evaluation

The patient has a vertical excess of the lower midface with excess dental and gingival show (Fig. 6-96).

Osteotomy

An upper buccal sulcus incision is made with subperiosteal dissection made over the zygomatic buttress at the level of the nasal floor and the lower part of the nasal septum. With a reciprocating saw, the predetermined thickness of bone slice is cut from either side of the maxilla. Care must be taken to cut the bone slice in a wedge shape with a thinner posterior part. A curved osteotome is used to separate the maxillary tuberosity and pterygoid plates. With a double-ball osteotome, a strip of the nasal septum is removed. The maxilla can now be repositioned. Rigid fixation is employed (Fig. 6-96).

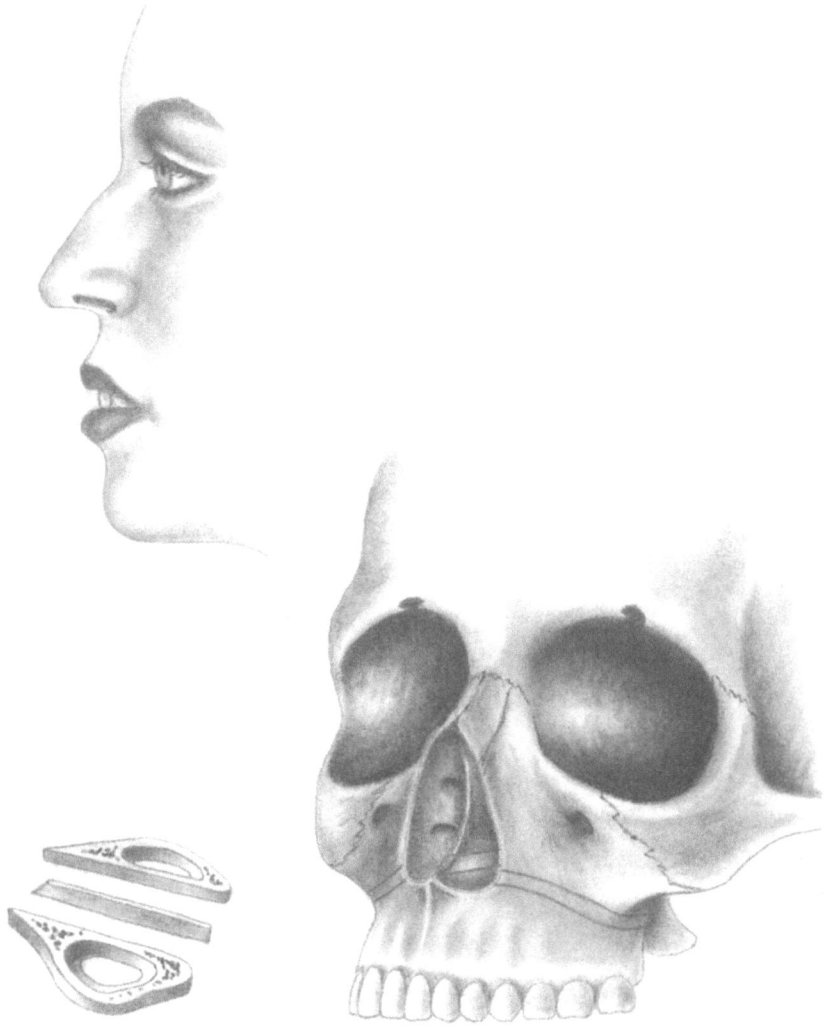

Figure 6–96

Preoperative Evaluation

On lateral view, the patient shows a short and retruded lower mid-face with a class III occlusion (Fig. 6-97).

Osteotomy

The osteotomy from a lower anterior to a high posterior position can be used for the treatment of this deformity. The procedure is similar to the low Le Fort I osteotomy. Care should be taken at the cuspid level since its root is significantly longer than molar roots. This osteotomy results in lengthening of the maxilla as it is moved forward (Fig. 6-97).

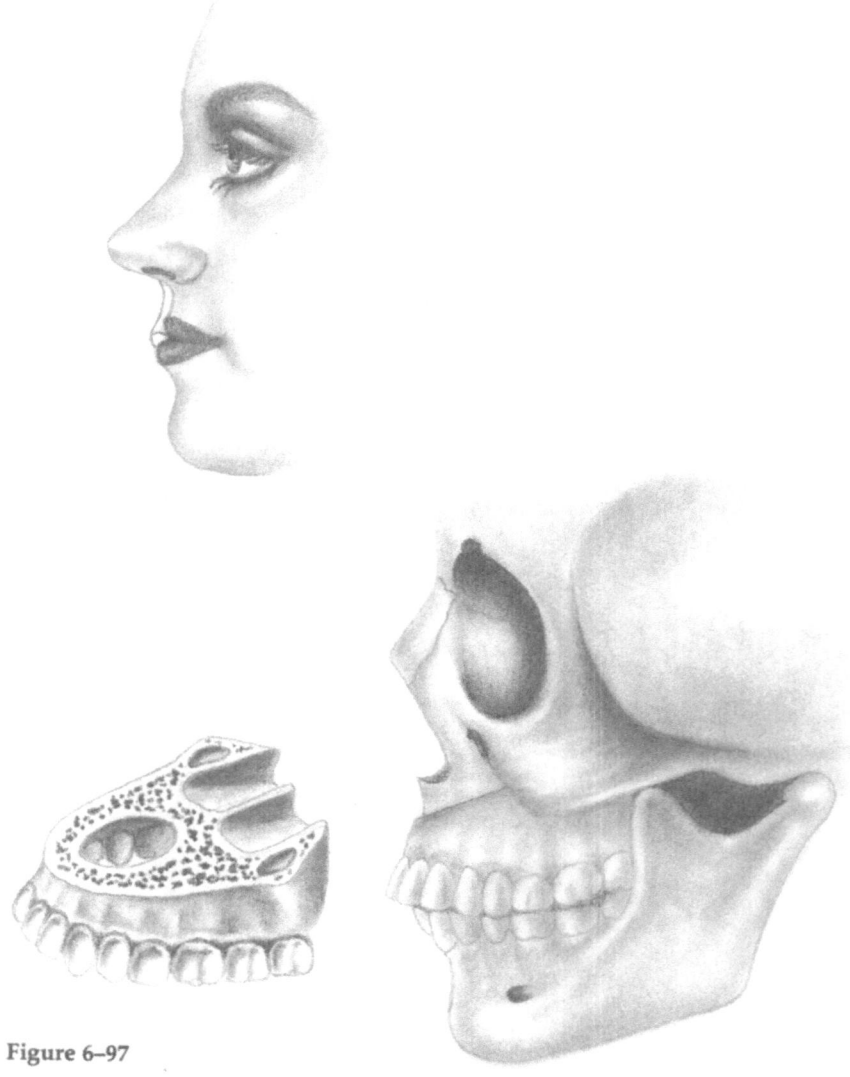

Figure 6–97

Preoperative Evaluation

This patient presents a midface retrusion involving the maxilla and the malar eminences. The patient has also a class III occlusion (Fig. 6-98).

Osteotomy

The lower blepharoplasty incision is made and the subperiosteal dissection is performed over the orbital floor, posteriorly to the inferior orbital fissure. With the orbital contents protected, the osteotomy directed to the inferior orbital fissure is made on the medial orbital floor. With a small reciprocating saw, the zygomatic arch is cut in an oblique direction. An upper buccal sulcus incision is made and the periosteum is elevated from the paranasal regions. An osteotomy is made from the piriform rim to the infraorbital rim and the pterygopalatine disjunction is completed by a curved osteotome. A double-ball osteotome is used to separate the nasal septum from the nasal floor. With Rowe disimpaction forceps, the down-fracture of the maxillomalar complex is done. The complex is advanced to the new position and rigid fixation is employed (Fig. 6-98).

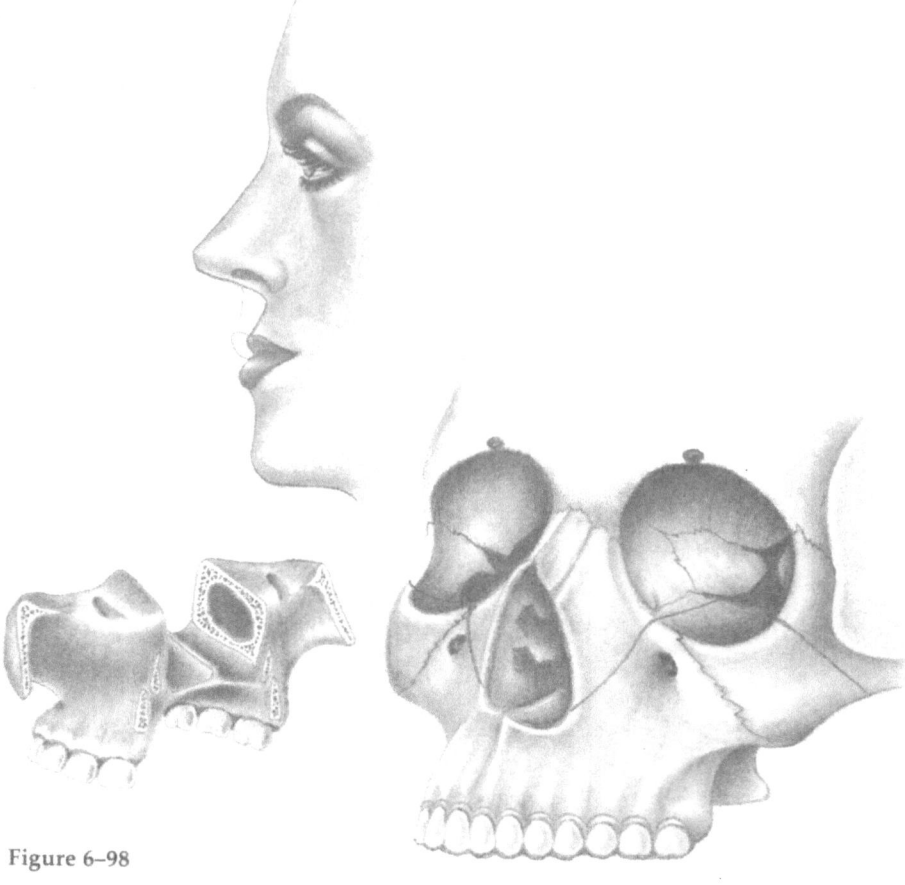

Figure 6–98

Preoperative Evaluation

This patient presents a retrusion of the maxilla with underdeveloped malar eminences and a class III occlusion (Fig. 6-99).

Osteotomy

The upper sulcus incision is made from first molar to first molar. The periosteum is elevated from the nasal floor, the zygomatic buttress, the front of the maxilla, and the paranasal regions. The lower blepharoplasty incision is used to expose the orbital rim and floor. With a reciprocating saw, the osteotomies are made on the front of the maxilla as shown. Using a short burr, an osteotomy is made on the orbital floor 5 mm from the orbital rim. The posterior part of the zygomatic buttress is separated by a curved saw. For pterygopalatine disjunction, a fine curved osteotome is employed and a double-ball osteotome is used to separate the nasal septum from the nasal floor. With Rowe disimpaction forceps, the down-fracture of the midface complex is carried out and pulled anteriorly. Rigid fixation is used (Fig. 6-99).

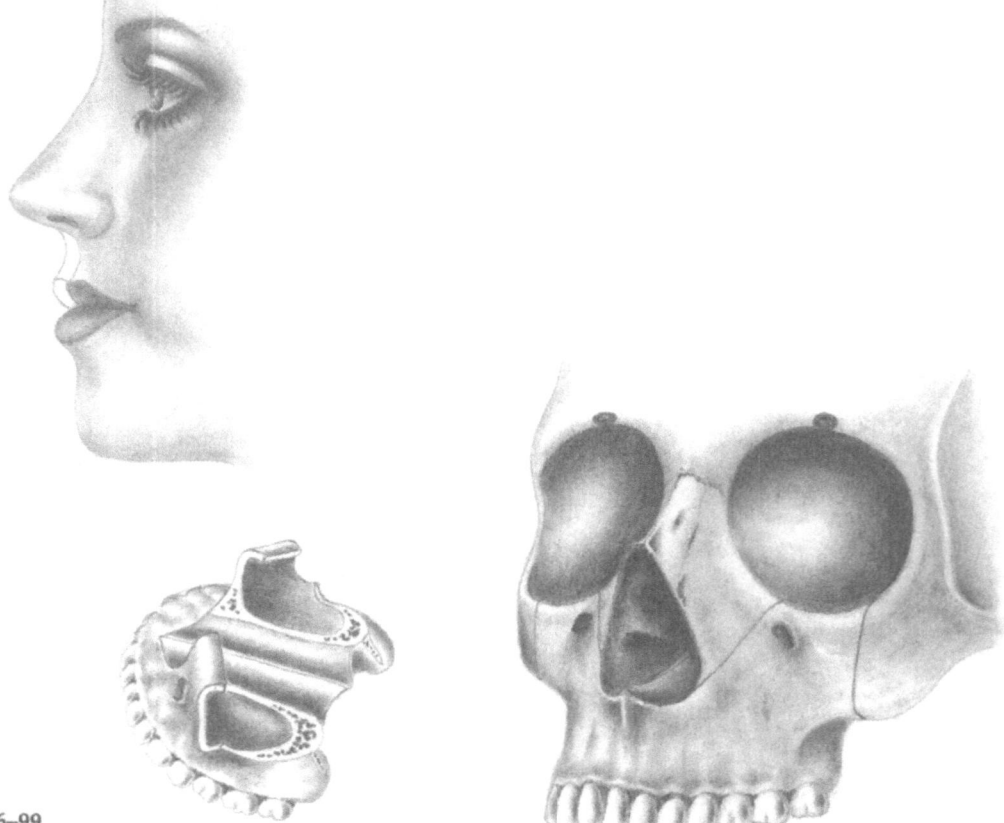

Figure 6–99

Preoperative Evaluation

The patient has a retrusion of the maxilla, the malar eminences, and the lateral orbital rims, as well as a class III occlusion (Fig. 6-100).

Osteotomy

The coronal incision is made and the subperiosteal dissection is performed over the medial orbital wall, the lateral orbital rim, and the zygomatic arch. With a small reciprocating saw, the osteotomy is made from the zygomatic arch to the lateral orbital wall and the inferior orbital fissure. With the orbital contents protected, the osteotomy is directed to the inferior orbital fissure on the paranasal region and the orbital floor. The pterygopalatine disjunction is completed via an intraoral stab wound. With a double-ball osteotome, the nasal septum is separated from the nasal floor via a small upper buccal sulcus incision. Rowe disimpaction forceps are used to down-fracture the maxillo-malar complex and to pull it to the new position. Rigid fixation is employed (Fig. 6-100).

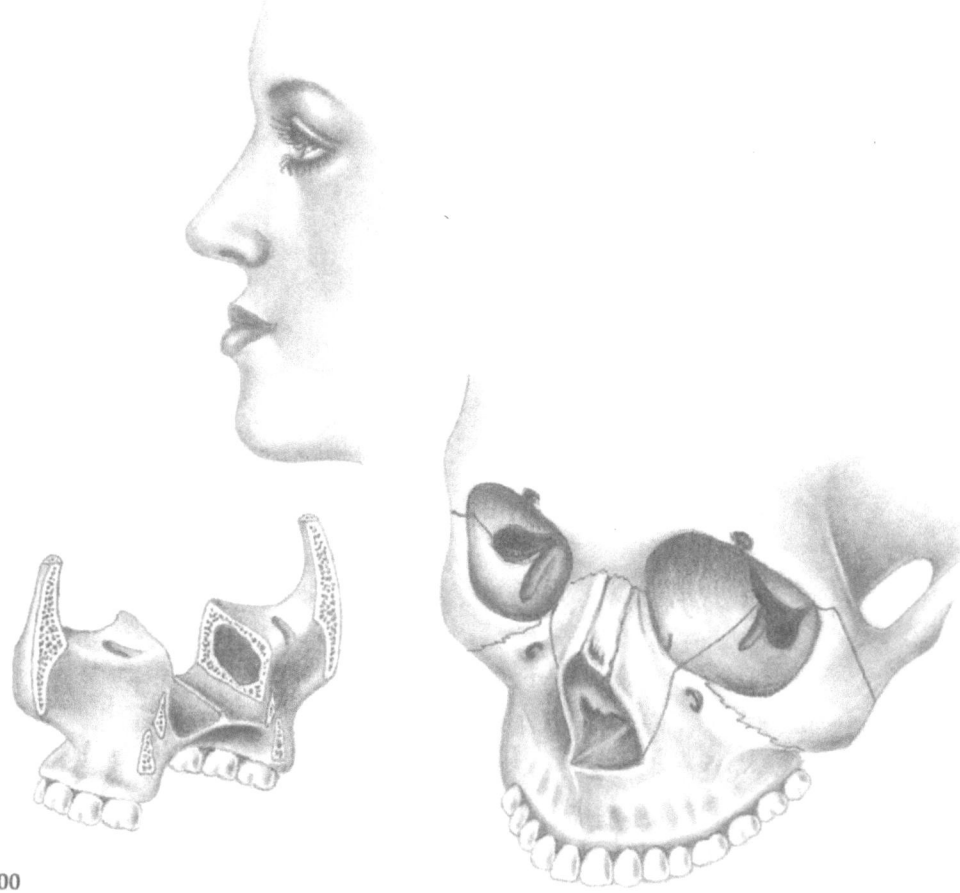

Figure 6–100

Preoperative Evaluation

The patient has a retrusion of the lower midface as well as a class III occlusion (Fig. 6-101).

Osteotomy

The upper buccal sulcus incision is made with subperiosteal dissection performed over the zygomatic buttress, nasal floor, and malar eminences. With a right-angle burr, a horizontal osteotomy is made 5 mm below the infraorbital rim. Using a curved osteotome, the medial sinus wall is cut vertically, anterior to the nasolacrimal tube. The posterior part of the maxilla is cut horizontally as shown. With a fine curved osteotome, the lateral sinus wall and the pterygopalatine junction is divided. This is done bilaterally. A double-ball osteotome is used to separate the nasal septum from the nasal floor and Rowe disimpaction forceps are employed to pull forward the midface complex (Fig. 6-101).

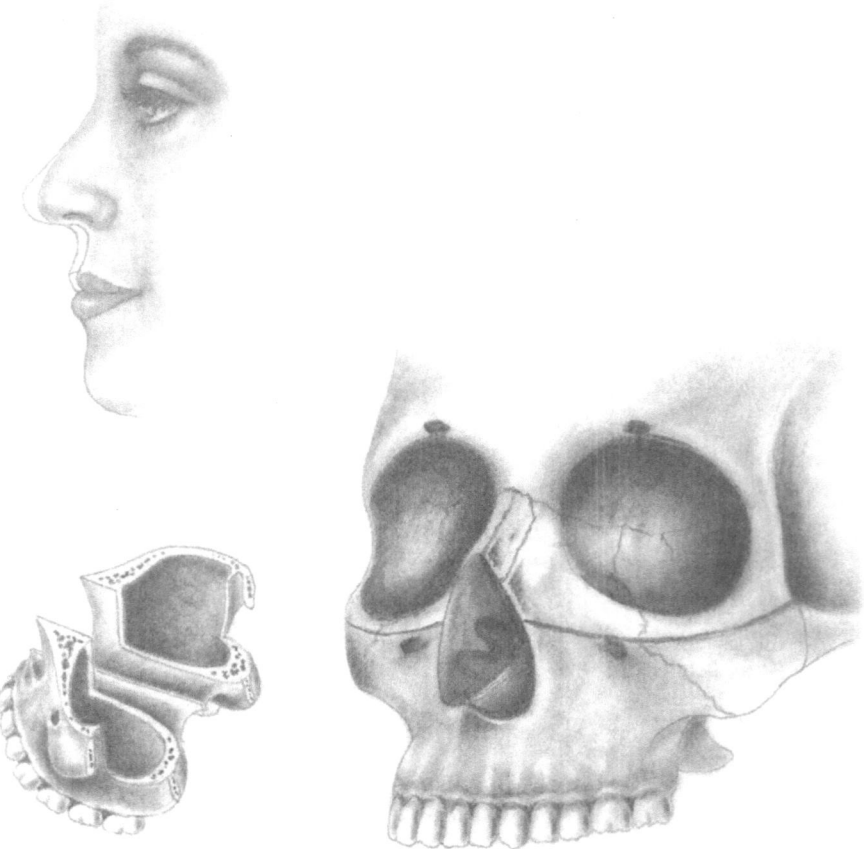

Figure 6–101

Preoperative Evaluation

This patient has a retrusion of the midface including the nose and the maxilla, but the malar eminences are well-developed. There is a class III occlusion (Fig. 6-102).

Osteotomy

The upper buccal sulcus incision is made to expose the maxilla, and the subperiosteal dissection is performed over the zygomatic buttress and the paranasal regions. The coronal incision is used to expose the nasal root and the medial orbital wall and floor. With a reciprocating saw, a horizontal osteotomy is made across the zygomatic buttress. The pterygopalatine junction is separated by a small curved osteotome. Care must be taken not to damage the maxillary artery and the pterygoid venous plexus. A double-ball osteotome is used to cut the nasal septum at the level of the nasal floor. Via the coronal incision, the nasal bone is transected at the level below the anterior ethmoidal foramen. With a fine osteotome, the medial orbital wall and floor osteotomy is made posterior to the lacrimal apparatus. An oblique cut is made from the inferior orbital rim to the maxillary osteotomy. Again, the double-ball osteotome is used to cut the nasal septum to meet the previous nasal septum cut. Now the nasomaxillary complex can be advanced to the new position and held with intermaxillary fixation. Miniplate fixation can be placed along the frontal osteotomy lines (Fig. 6-102).

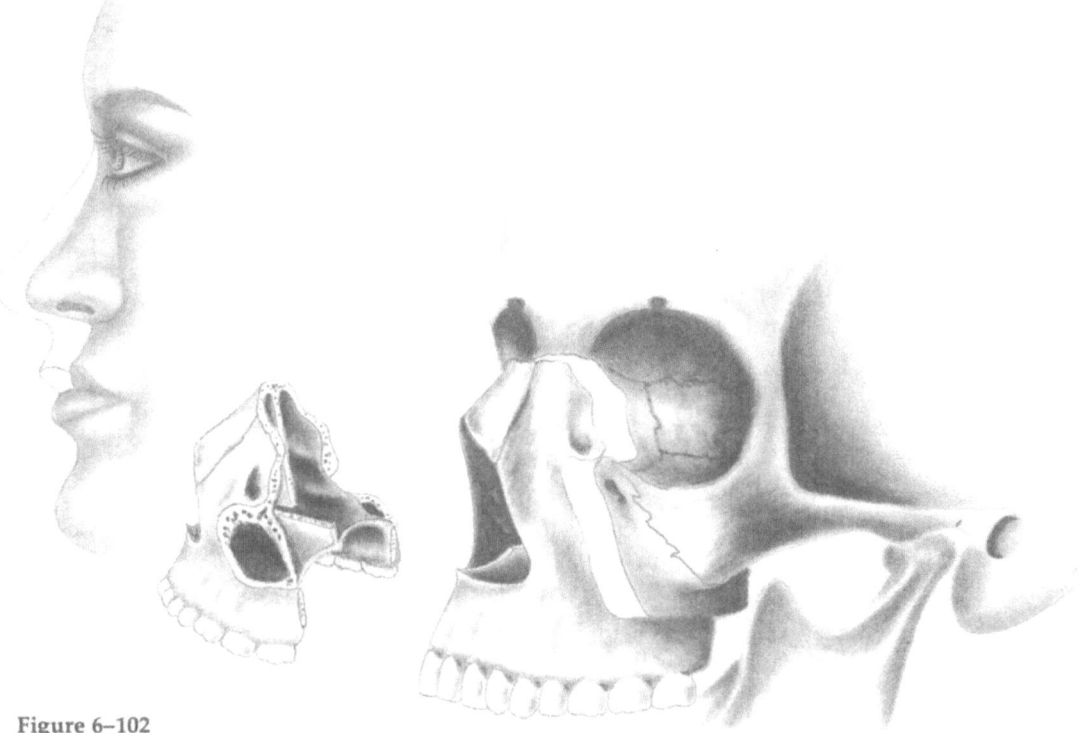

Figure 6–102

Preoperative Evaluation

The patient shows a retrusion of the midface involving the nasal bridge and the maxilla. The malar eminences are prominent. The patient also has a class III occlusion (Fig. 6-103).

Osteotomy

A coronal incision is used for the exposure with the subperiosteal dissection performed over the nasal bridge, the zygomatic arches, and the malar eminences. With the orbital contents protected, the osteotomy is made sagittally across the maxillary sinus, followed by an osteotomy directed to the inferior orbital fissure on the medial orbital wall. Via the temporal fossa, the pterygopalatine disjunction is carried out using a fine curved osteotome. The same procedure is performed bilaterally. The frontonasal osteotomy is made below the level of the anterior ethmoidal foramen, and a double-ball osteotome is employed to divide the nasal septum from the cranial base. Using Rowe disimpaction forceps, the midface complex is pulled forward (Fig. 6-103).

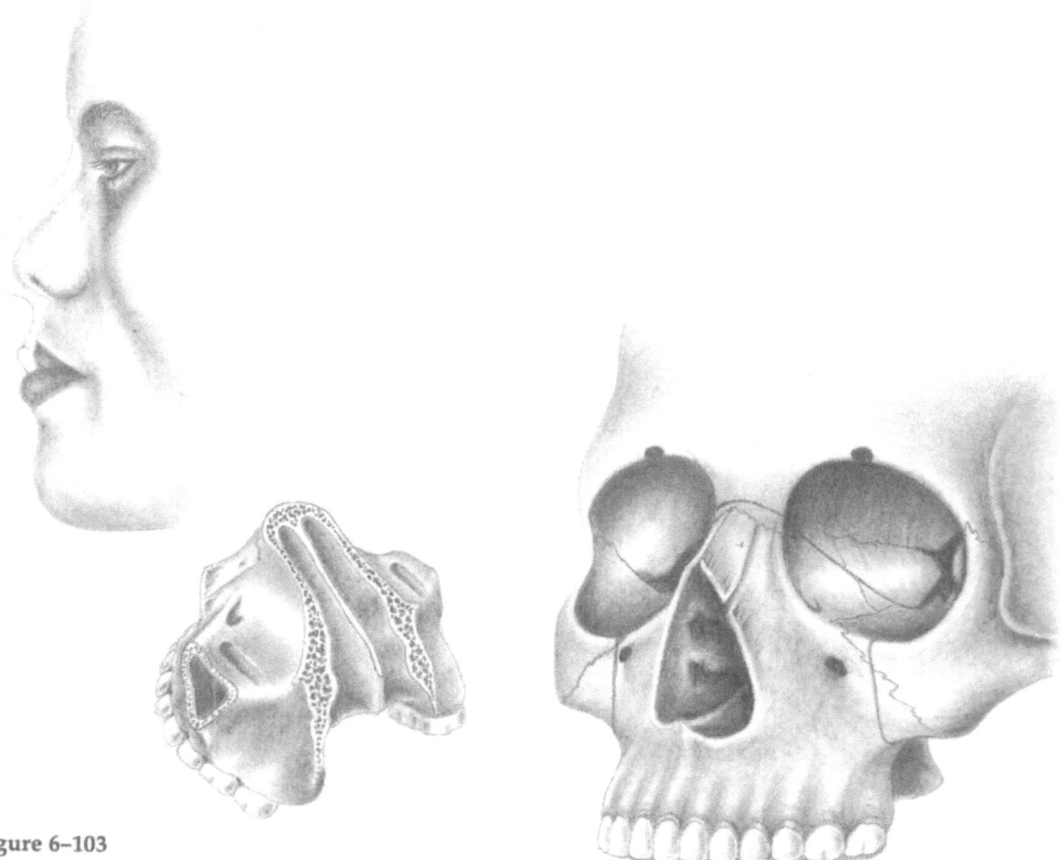

Figure 6–103

Preoperative Evaluation

The patient has an upper midface retrusion involving the nose, malar eminences, and lateral orbital rims. The occlusion is ideal (Fig. 6-104).

Osteotomy

A coronal incision is made and the subperiosteal dissection is performed over the nasal bridge, the lateral orbital rim, and the zygomatic arch. The anterior two-thirds of the temporal muscle is elevated from its fossa. The dissection is continued to the inferior orbital fissure. The zygomatic arch is cut. With a small reciprocating saw, the lateral sinus wall, the orbital floor, and the lateral orbital wall are cut in a cephalad direction. With a curved saw, an osteotomy is made on the medial orbital wall behind the lacrimal groove to meet the previous osteotomy on the orbital floor. An upper buccal sulcus incision is made with subperiosteal dissection performed over the nasal floor and the lateral wall of the nasal cavity. Using a fine curved osteotome, the medial sinus wall is cut vertically, posterior to the nasolacrimal tube. With an oscillating saw, a horizontal osteotomy is made at the level of the nasal floor. A double-ball osteotome is employed to separate the nasal septum from the nasal floor. The frontonasal osteotomy is then made below the level of the anterior ethmoidal foramen. The double-ball osteotome is used to divide the nasal septum from the cranial base and an elevator is employed to raise the midface complex (Fig. 6-104).

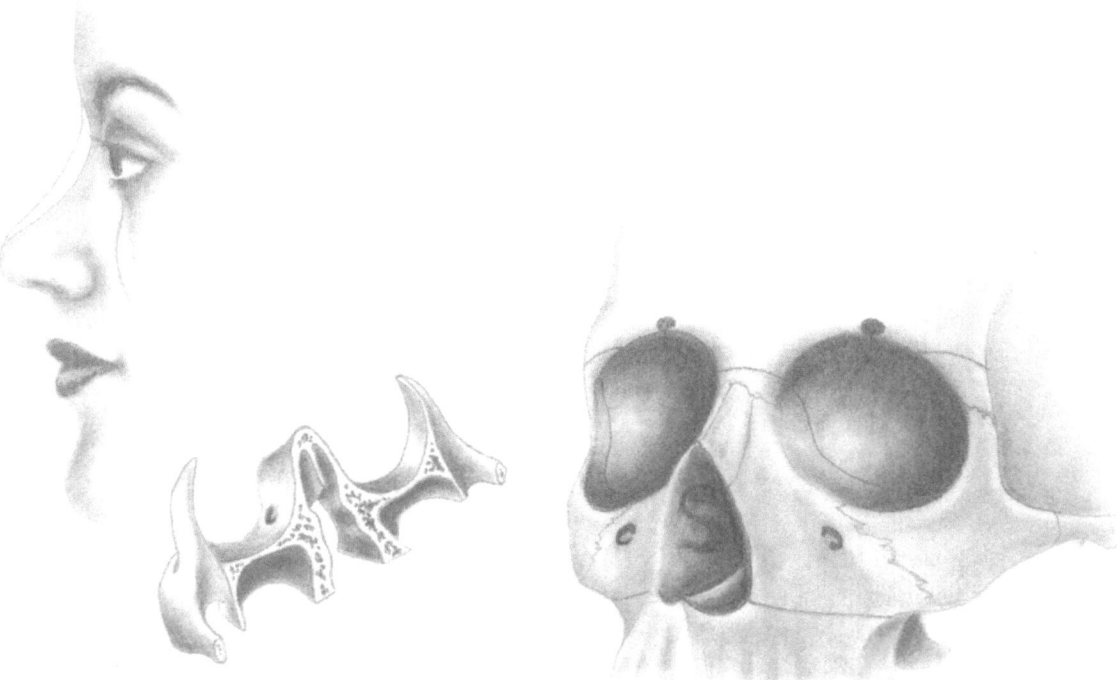

Figure 6–104

Preoperative Evaluation

The patient has a retrusion of the midface involving the nasal bridge, the malar eminences, and the lateral orbital rims, as well as a class III occlusion (Fig. 6-105).

Osteotomy

The osteotomies of the nasal bridge, the zygomatic arches, the lateral orbital walls, the medial orbital walls, and the orbital floors are the same as the previous case. The canthus must be left attached to the bone block, which will be moved later. The upper buccal sulcus incision is made with the subperiosteal dissection performed over the nasal floor and the pterygopalatine junction. With a curved saw, the posterior part of the zygomatic buttress is cut. The pterygopalatine disjunction is accomplished using a fine curved osteotome. Rowe disimpaction forceps are used to perform a down-fracture of the midface complex. The separation of the midface is completed by a gently rocking and twisting motion. The midface complex is advanced to the preplanned position and the bone grafts are inserted into the gaps. Intermaxillary and rigid fixation are employed (Fig. 6-105).

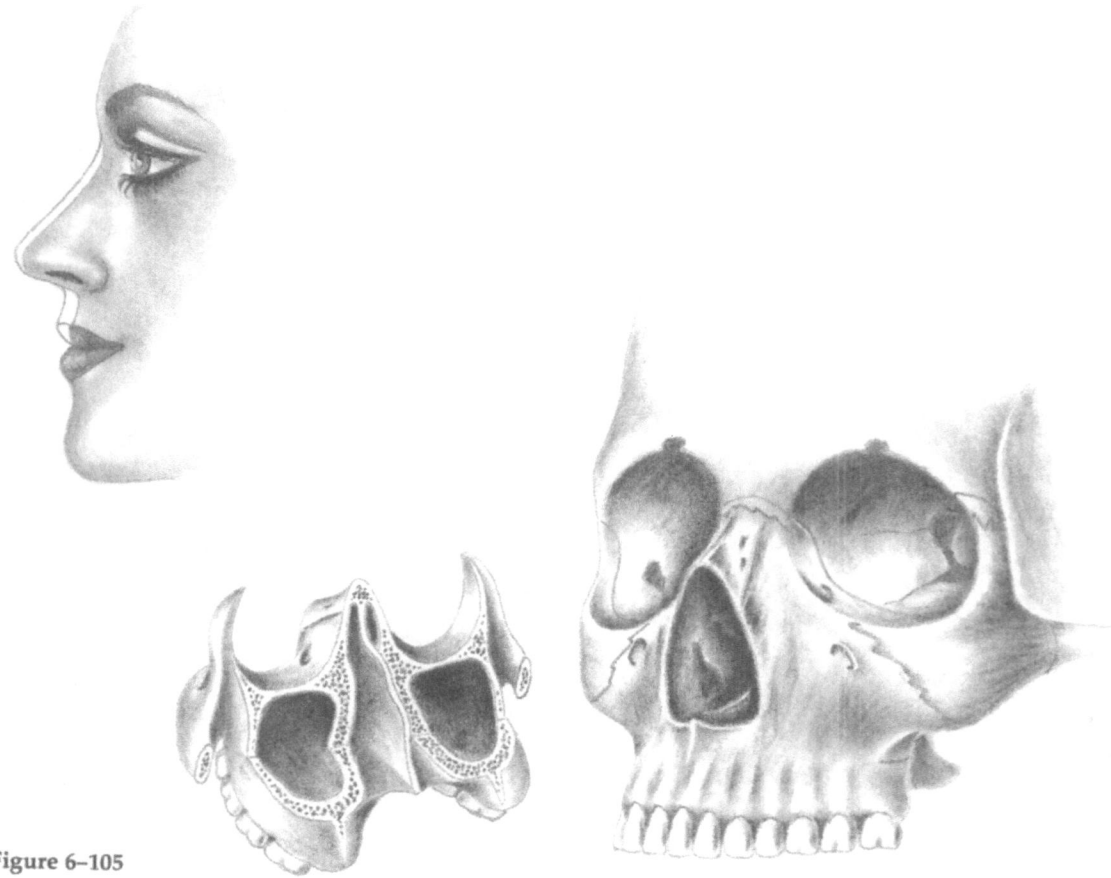

Figure 6–105

Preoperative Evaluation

This patient presents a midface retrusion as well as a class III occlusion (Fig. 6-106).

Osteotomy

Exposure is provided via a coronal incision. The facial soft tissue is elevated subperiosteally from the orbital rims, the front of the maxilla, the nasal bridge, and the zygomatic arches. The anterior two-thirds of the temporal muscle is elevated from its fossa. The dissection is performed down to the inferior orbital fissure and the pterygopalatine junction. Using a reciprocating saw, an osteotomy is made from the inferior orbital fissure to the lateral orbital wall and the zygomatic arch. With the orbital contents protected, the osteotomy is directed to the inferior orbital fissure on the medial orbital wall. The pterygopalatine dissection is done by a fine curved osteotome via the temporal fossa. The procedure is repeated on the opposite side. The frontonasal osteotomy is made below the level of the anterior ethmoidal foramen. A double-ball osteotome is used to separate the nasal septum from the cranial base. With Rowe disimpaction forceps, the down-fracture of the midface complex is made and pulled forward to the predetermined position. Rigid fixation is employed (Fig. 6-106).

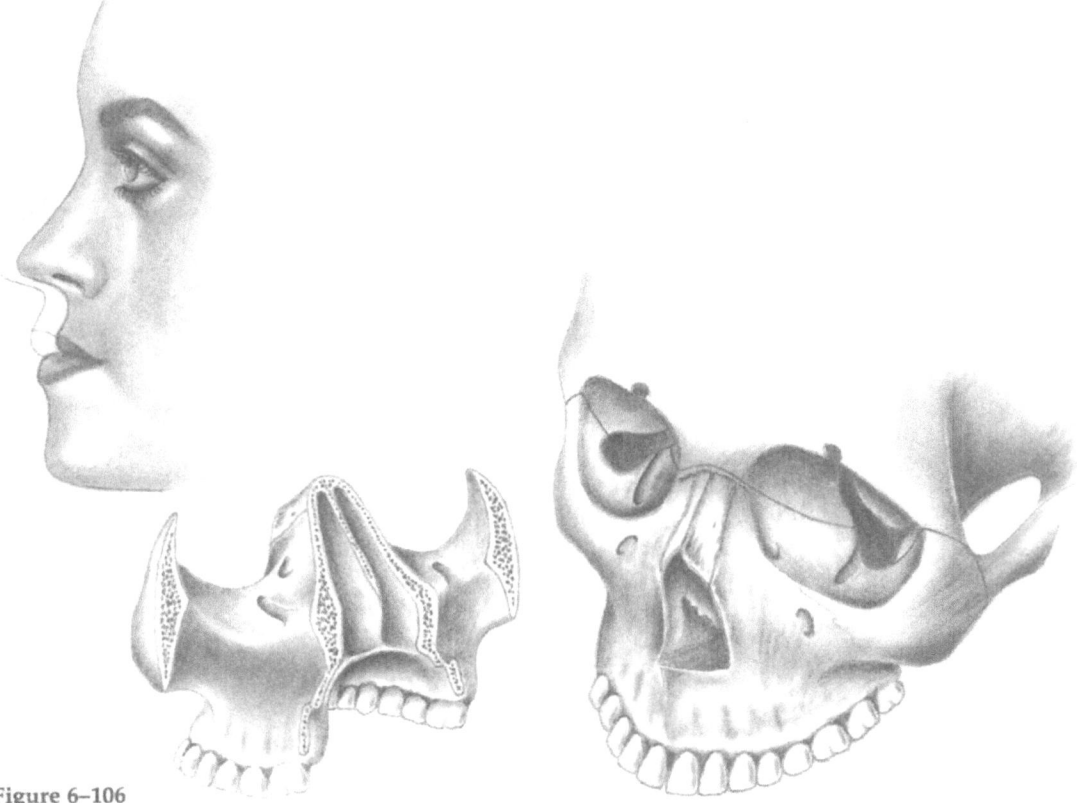

Figure 6–106

Preoperative Evaluation

On lateral view, this patient presents a vertical excess of the lower midface with excess dental and gingival show in repose (Fig. 6-107).

Osteotomy

A lower Le Fort I osteotomy is performed. The maxillary osteotomy is made horizontally at a level at least 6 mm above the dental apices. The predetermined bone on the maxilla is removed with a burr or a reciprocating saw. The segment is repositioned and rigid fixation is used. Overcorrection should be avoided. If the bone removed is more than 4–5 mm in thickness, a standard Le Fort I osteotomy is an alternative (Fig. 6-107).

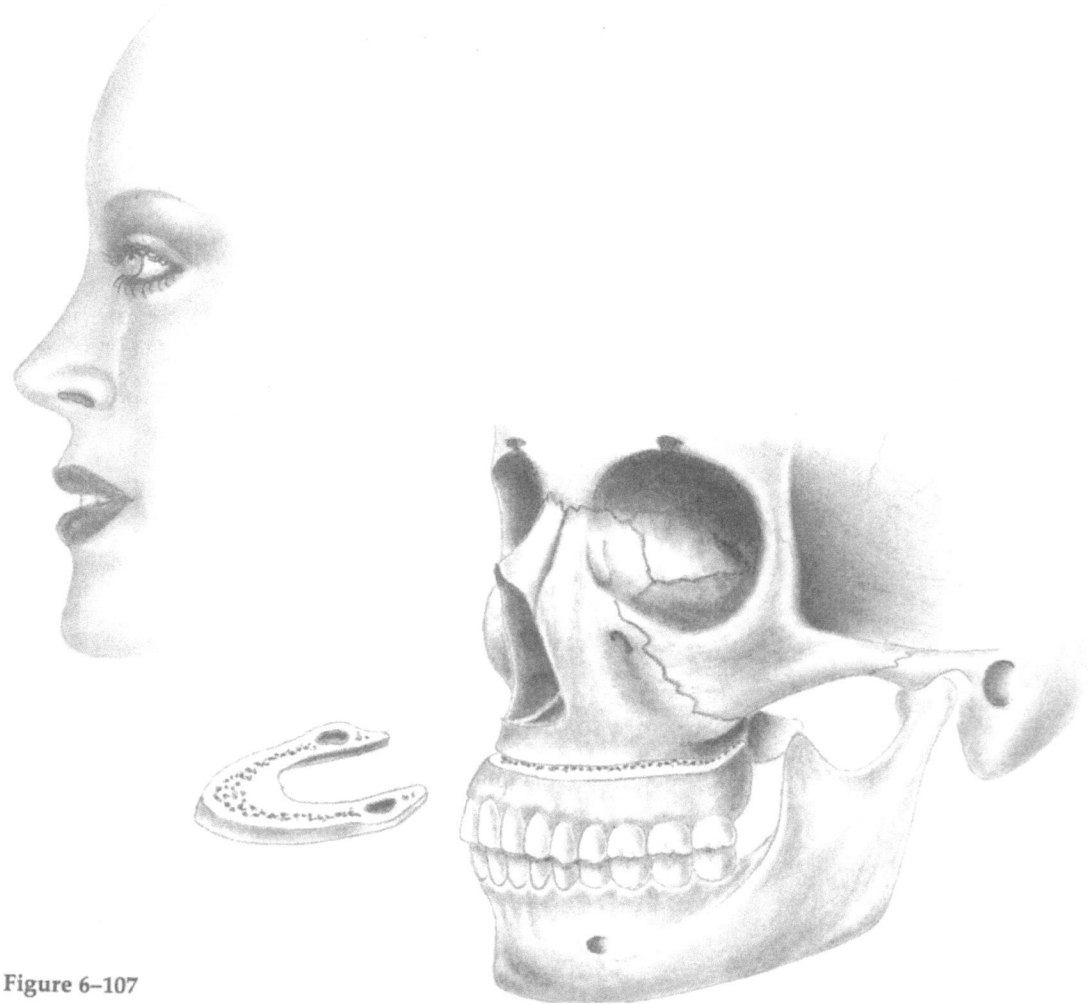

Figure 6–107

Mandibular Region

Preoperative Evaluation

The patient has an overjet occlusion, but the relationship between the chin and the maxilla is ideal. The lower facial height is normal (Fig. 6-108).

Osteotomy

A modified mandibular sagittal split osteotomy is performed. The posterior buccal fat pad mucosal incision is used for the exposure. The osteotomy is made along the external oblique line of the mandible and down to the midportion of the mandibular body. The procedure is performed bilaterally. A lower buccal sulcus incision is made medially, and a horizontal osteotomy is performed 4 mm below the mental foramen. A small hand saw is used to cut the medial portions on both ascending mandibular rami. The segment is advanced to obtain a normal occlusion. Intermaxillary and rigid fixation are used. The advantage of this osteotomy is there is no manipulation of the temporomandibular joint function (Fig. 6-108).

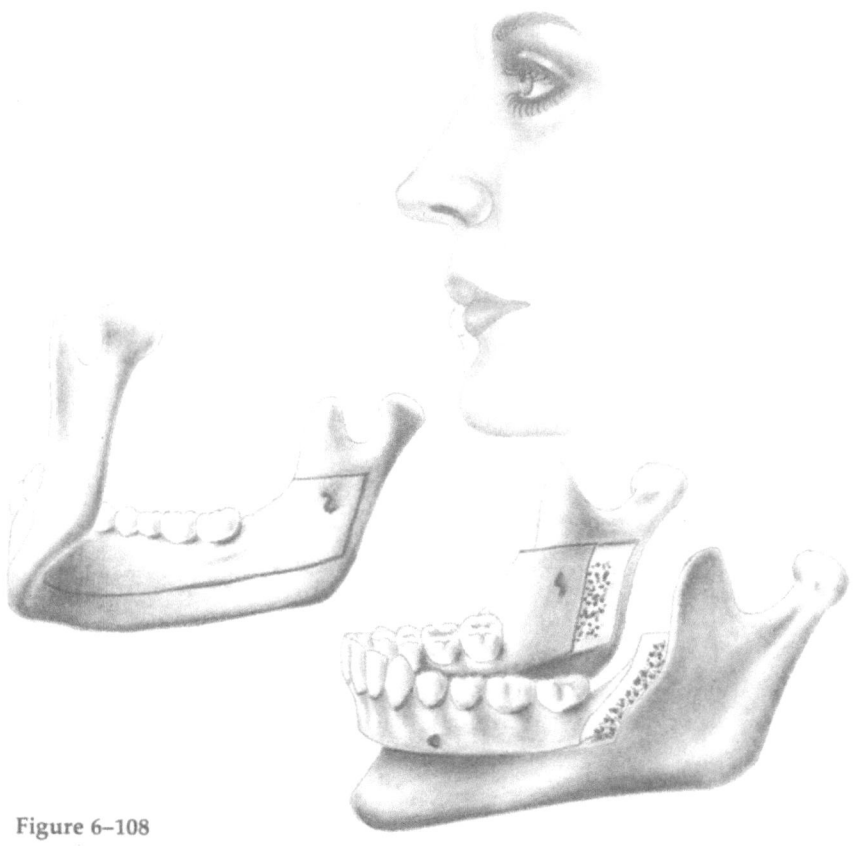

Figure 6–108

Preoperative Evaluation

The patient demonstrates a horizontal deficiency of the chin. The occlusion is normal (Fig. 6-109).

Osteotomy

The vertical chin split osteotomy can be used for treating this deformity. A lower buccal sulcus incision is made lateral to the first premolar on either side. Subperiosteal dissection is performed vertically on the both ends of the incision. Care must be taken to prevent injuring the mental nerve. By placing the reciprocating saw vertically before the mental foramen, an osteotomy is made around the chin. While the osteotomy is being performed, the surgeon's left index finger is placed on the inframandibular rim to palpate the saw tip. The segment is advanced and the bone graft is inserted into the gap. Two or three longer screws are used for the fixation. Some advantages with this osteotomy include (1) minimal disturbance of the intraoral structure, (2) more advancement, (3) improved frontal contour, (4) more bone contact, and (5) easy fixation. The disadvantages are the need for a well-executed procedure and the need for a bone graft (Fig. 6-109).

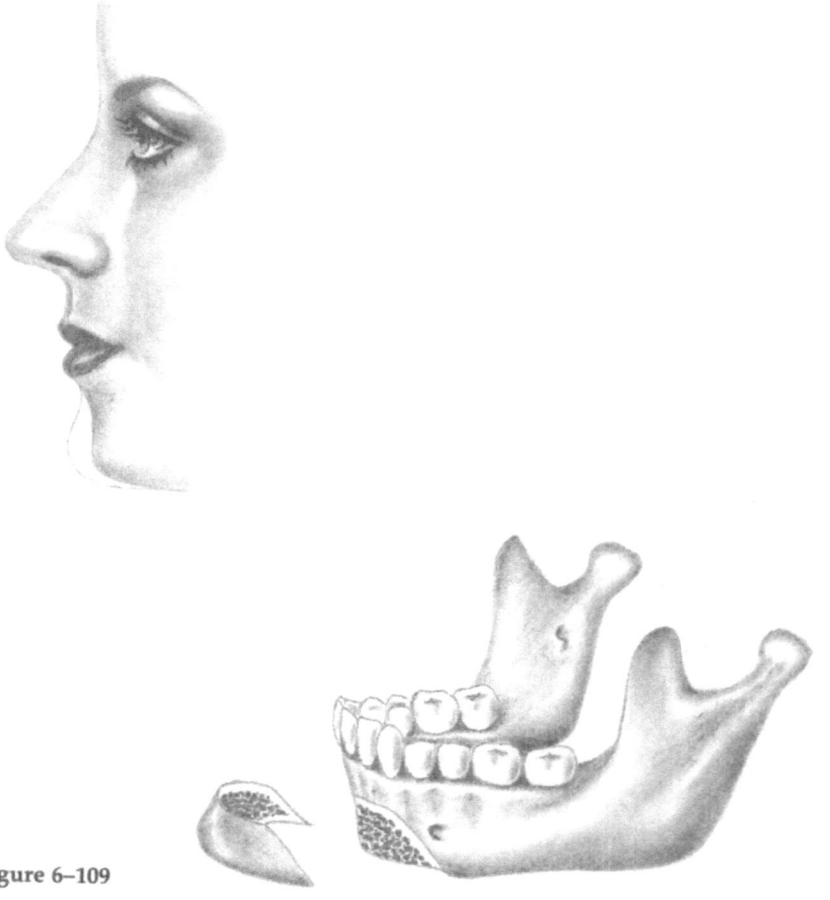

Figure 6–109

Preoperative Evaluation

The frontal mandibular teeth are inclined anteriorly and overerupted. The relationship between the maxilla and the chin is ideal (Fig. 6-110).

Osteotomy

Usually the first mandibular premolar is extracted on either side. A wedge-shaped bone block is cut 6 mm below the dental apices as shown. With a fine burr, a wedge-shaped bone block is removed from the area below the extracted premolar bilaterally and the segment is rotated posteriorly. Care must be taken to prevent injuring the inferior alveolar nerve. Before using rigid fixation, intermaxillary fixation is employed to obtain an ideal occlusion (Fig. 6-110).

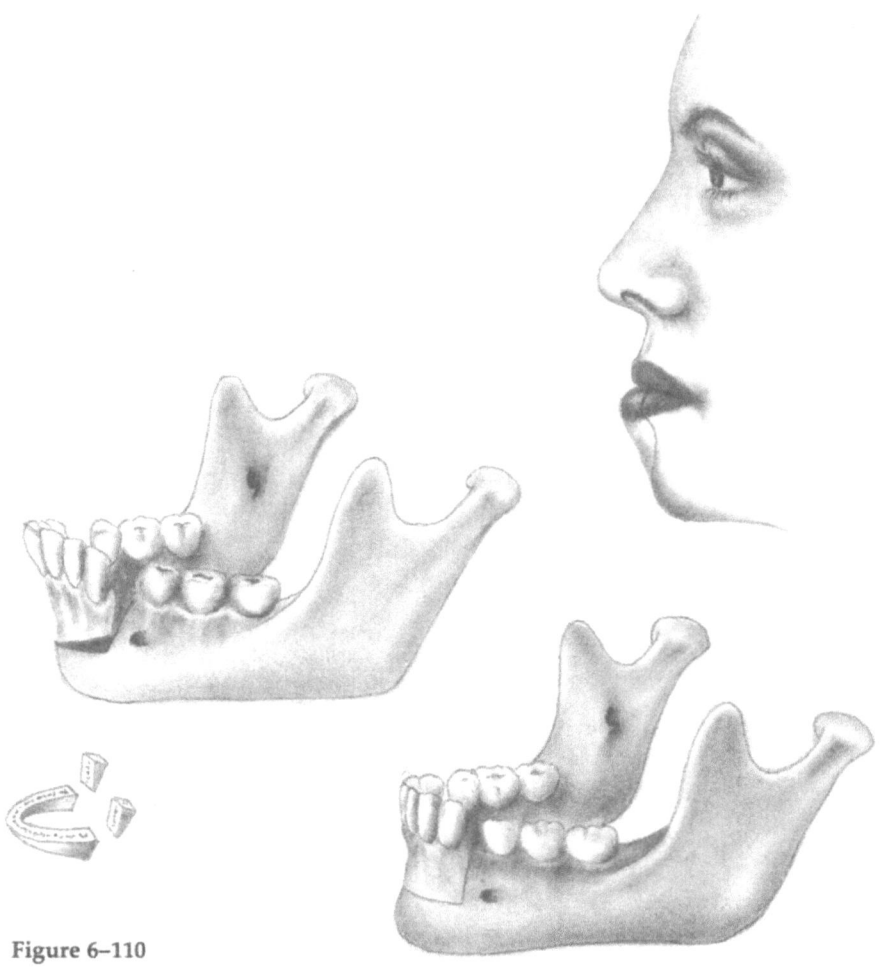

Figure 6–110

Preoperative Evaluation

This patient has a class III occlusion. The chin is well balanced with respect to the face (Fig. 6-111).

Osteotomy

The first mandibular premolar is extracted on either side. With an oscillating saw, a horizontal osteotomy is made 4 mm below the mental foramen via a lower buccal sulcus incision. A small oval burr is used to remove the alveolar bone of the first mandibular premolar. Care must be taken not to damage the inferior alveolar nerve. Following the completion of the osteotomies, the segment can be retracted to the new position and rigid fixation is used. A burr can be used to smooth the step deformity on the anterior portion of the mandible (Fig. 6-111).

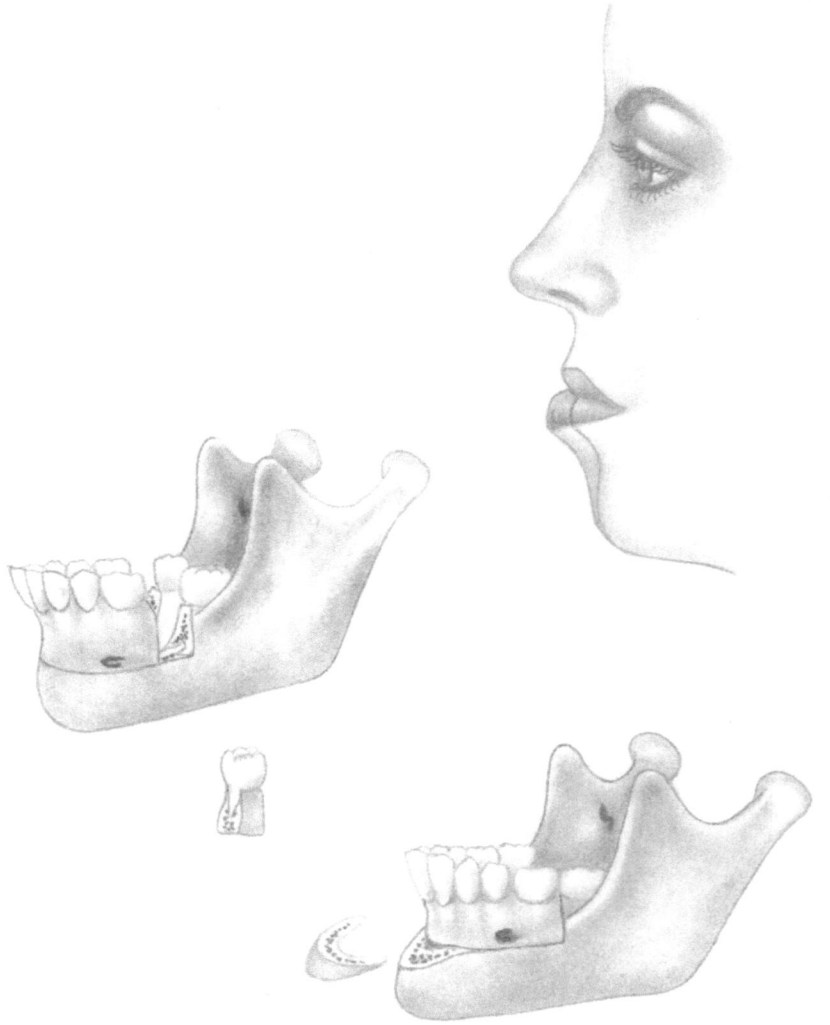

Figure 6–111

Preoperative Evaluation

This patient presents a class III occlusion and the relationship between the chin and the maxilla is ideal (Fig. 6-112).

Osteotomy

A modified mandibular sagittal split osteotomy can be used in this case. The posterior buccal fat pad mucosal incision is made halfway up the anterior margin of the ramus, and the periosteum is separated from the medial ramus. Using as oscillating saw, an initial medial horizontal osteotomy is performed 2 mm above the mandibular foramen. An osteotomy is made along the external oblique line of the mandible and down to the midportion of the mandibular body. The same procedure is performed on the contralateral side. A lower buccal sulcus incision is made medially and subperiosteal dissection is made around the incision. An osteotomy is carried horizontally at the level of 2 mm below the mental canals using an oscillating saw. Using a small hand saw, an osteotomy is made from medial to lateral to meet the osteotomy along the external oblique line bilaterally. The segment can now be retropositioned and fixed (Fig. 6-112).

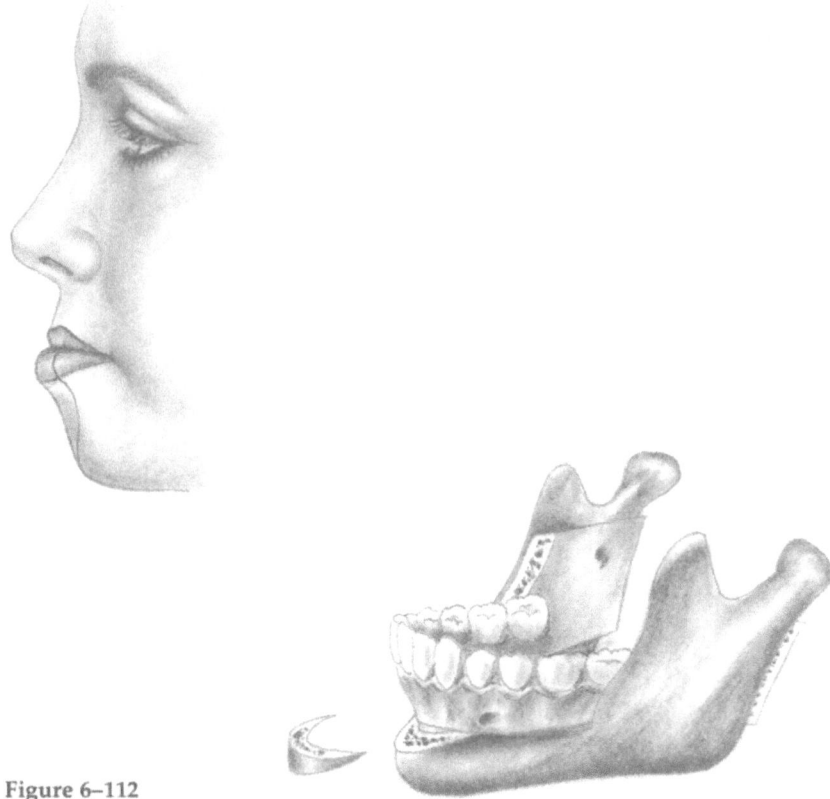

Figure 6–112

Preoperative Evaluation

This patient has retrognathia with an overjet occlusion. The relationships among the other parts of the face are normal (Fig. 6-113).

Osteotomy

A standard mandibular sagittal split osteotomy can be used for the treatment of this deformity. The posterior buccal fat pad mucosal incision is made and the periosteum of the medial ramus is separated by a periosteal elevator. Half of the full thickness of the ascending ramus is cut above the level of the mandibular foramen. With an oscillating saw blade, an osteotomy along the external oblique line and down to the inferior edge of the mandible is made to split the mandible into medial and lateral portions. The same procedure is done on the contralateral side of the mandible. The body of the mandible can now be advanced. Before the intermaxillary and rigid fixations are employed, make sure that the condylar head is seated in the glenoid fossa (Fig. 6-113).

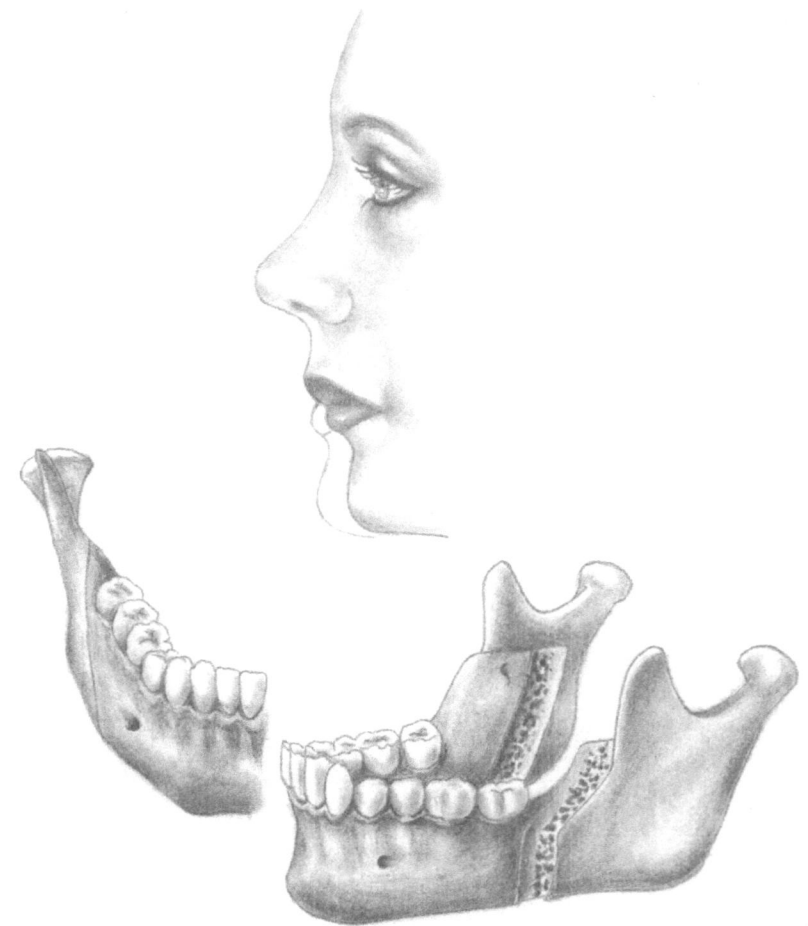

Figure 6–113

Preoperative Evaluation

This patient has a slightly retruded chin as well as an open-bite occlusion (Fig. 6-114).

Osteotomy

The incision is made in the cheek mucosa far laterally and halfway up the anterior margin of the ramus, avoiding exposure of the buccal fat pad. The subperiosteal dissection is made on the medial ramus and the inferior alveolar neurovascular bundle is identified. With an oscillating saw, an initial horizontal medial osteotomy is carried out 2 mm above the mandibular foramen. An osteotomy along the external oblique line and down to the inferior border of the mandible is made, splitting the mandible into a lateral and a medial portion. Once the osteotomies have been performed bilaterally, the mandible is rotated into its new position. At the time of performing rigid fixation, the condyle must be secured in the glenoid fossa with a bone clamp (Fig. 6-114).

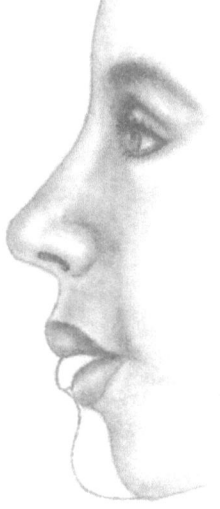

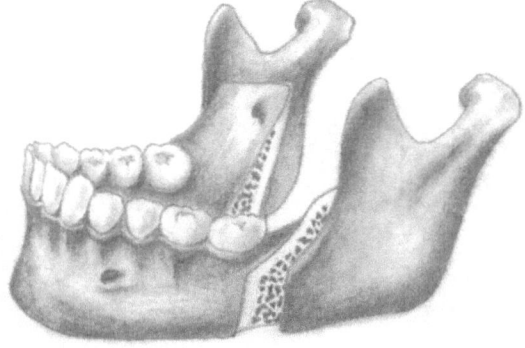

Figure 6–114

Preoperative Evaluation

The patient has a combined occlusal deformity with an open-bite and a class III occlusion. In addition, the patient has a vertical deficiency of the chin (Fig. 6-115).

Osteotomy

A modified mandibular sagittal split osteotomy is performed. The intermaxillary fixation is made by wiring the segment of the mandible to the maxilla. A bone graft is inserted into the gap to increase the vertical height of the chin, and rigid fixation is employed (Fig. 6-115).

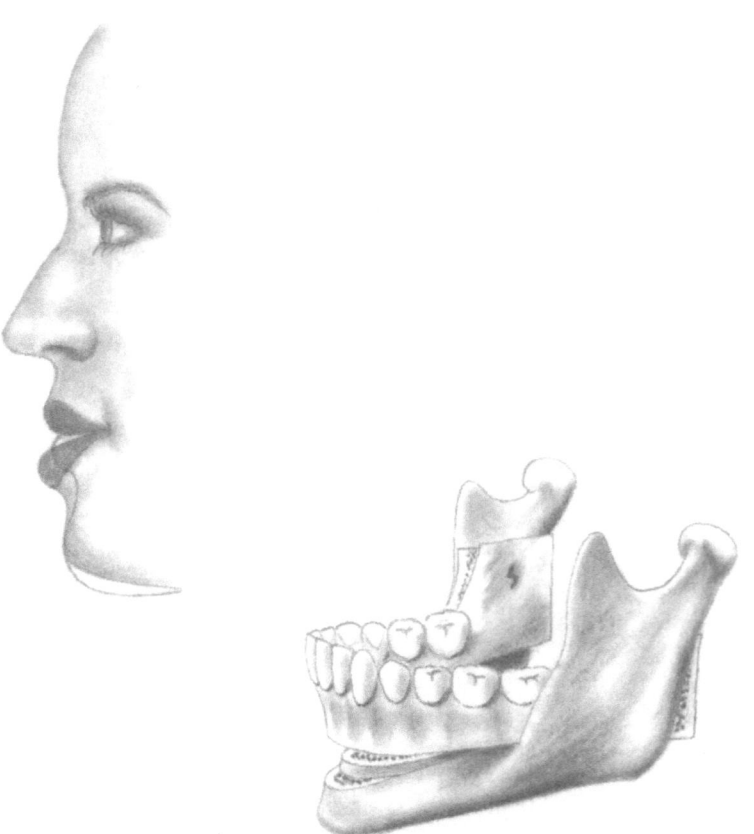

Figure 6–115

Preoperative Evaluation

On lateral view, the patient has a combined chin deformity with vertical excess and slight horizontal deficiency (Fig. 6-116).

Osteotomy

The approach is through a lower buccal sulcus incision. With an oscillating saw, two osteotomies are made on the chin according to the profile x-ray film. A wedge-shaped segment is removed. Two screws are used for fixation of the caudal segment (Fig. 6-116).

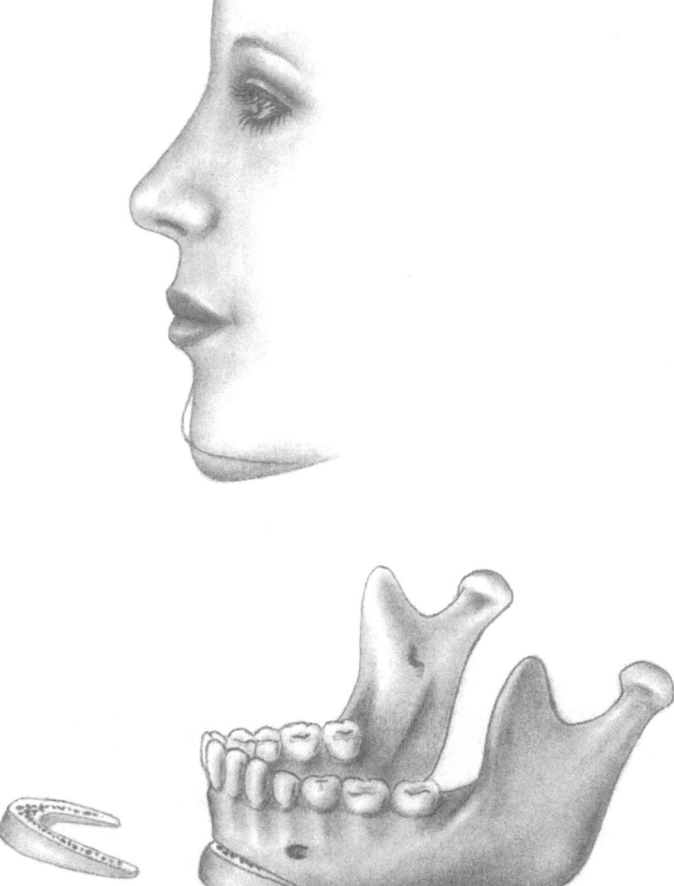

Figure 6–116

Preoperative Evaluation

The patient has a chin deformity with vertical excess and significant horizontal deficiency. The occlusion is ideal (Fig. 6-117).

Osteotomy

An incision is made on the lingual side of the lower buccal sulcus. The subperiosteal dissection is made down to the inferior mandibular rim. Two parallel cuts about 5 mm apart are made posteriorly and caudally and the segments are advanced the predetermined distance and secured with rigid fixation. Care must be taken to design the proper osteotomy orientation for the horizontal augment and the vertical reduction (Fig. 6-117).

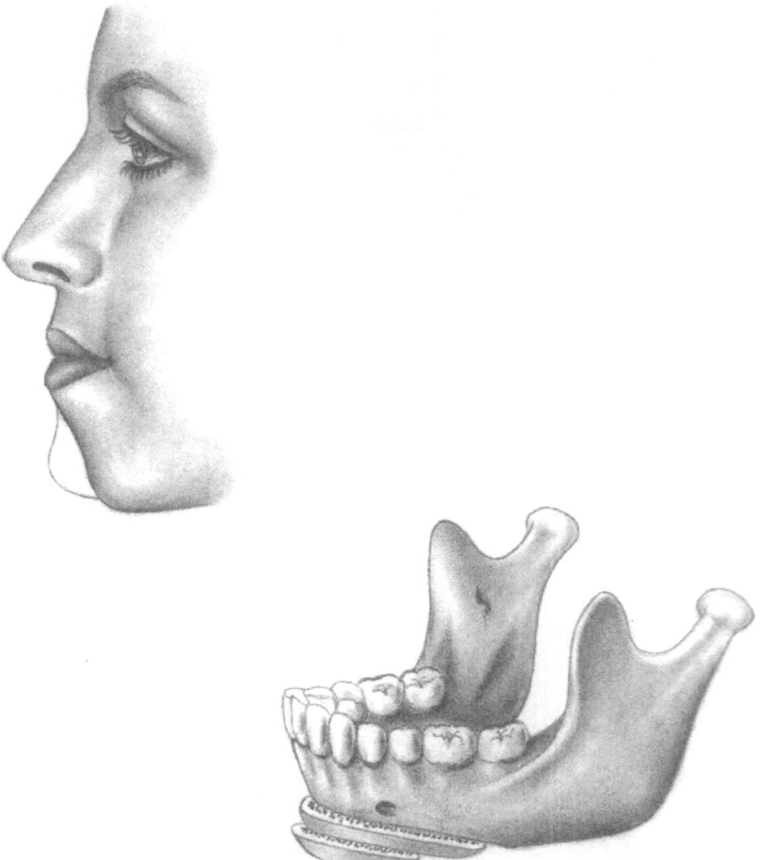

Figure 6–117

Preoperative Evaluation

On lateral view, the patient shows a significant horizontal excess of the chin, but the vertical height is ideal (Fig. 6-118).

Osteotomy

A lower buccal sulcus incision is used and the periosteum is elevated down to the inferior mandibular margin. With an oscillating saw, a horizontal osteotomy is made 6 mm below the dental apices. A small oval burr is used to remove a piece of bone from the lateral inferior margin of the chin bilaterally. The segment is retracted and rigid fixation is employed (Fig. 6-118).

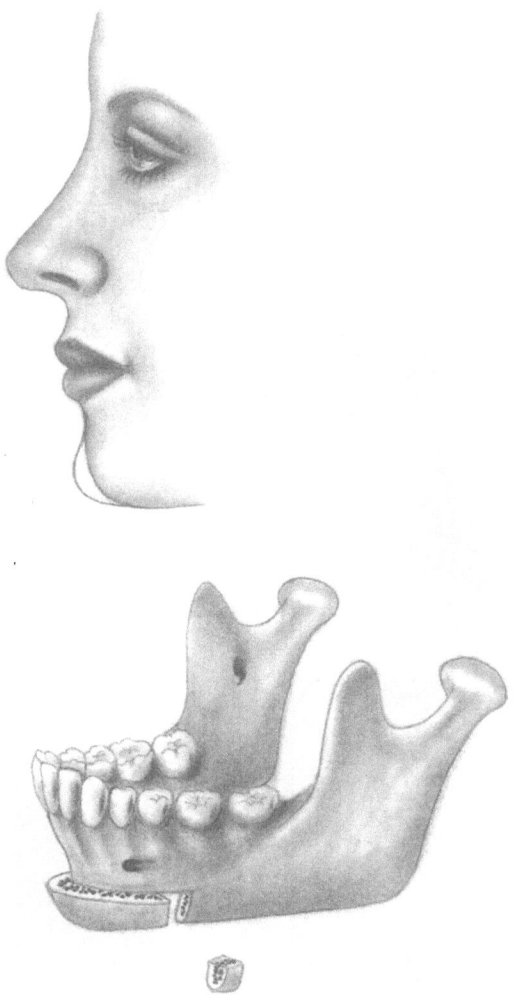

Figure 6–118

Preoperative Evaluation

On lateral view, this patient shows a retrusion of the chin with normal occlusion (Fig. 6-119).

Osteotomy

The bone graft for chin augmentation can be harvested from the cranial, rib, or iliac bone, and it is contoured into the predesigned shape. A lower buccal sulcus incision is made with the periosteum elevated from the mental surface and the bone graft is inserted. Two screws are used for fixation. To avoid a "witch chin," the periosteum should be fixed to the bone graft (Fig. 6-119).

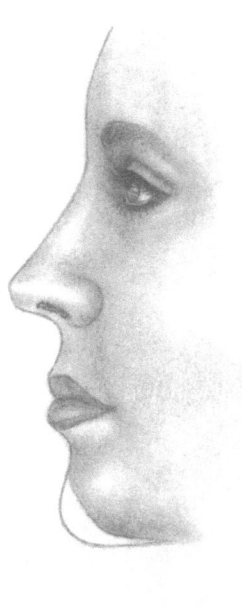

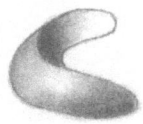

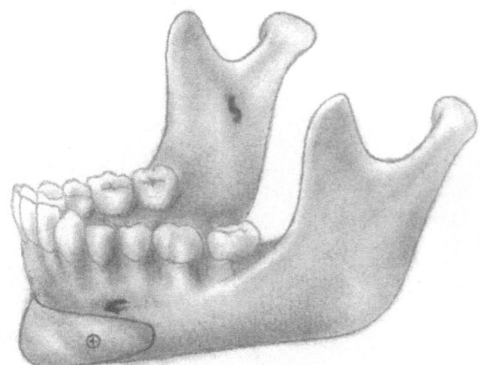

Figure 6–119

Preoperative Evaluation

The patient has a combined chin deformity with vertical excess and horizontal deficiency. The occlusion is normal (Fig. 6-120).

Osteotomy

A lower buccal sulcus incision is made and the subperiosteal dissection is performed. The soft tissue attachment to the chin should be preserved as much as possible. The osteotomy is directed caudally and posteriorly. Following completion of the osteotomy, the segment is moved anteriorly and cephalad. Rigid fixation is applied (Fig. 6-120).

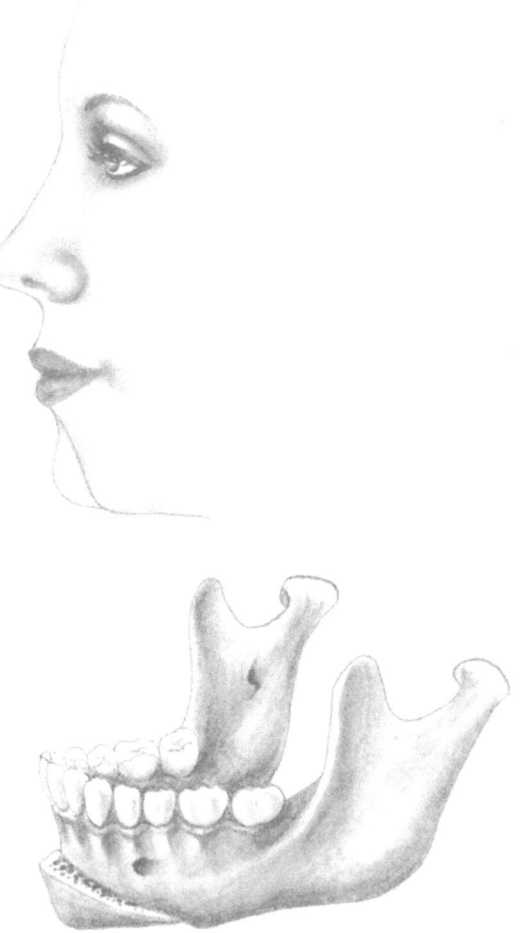

Figure 6–120

Preoperative Evaluation

The patient demonstrates a vertical macrogenia. Usually these patients have a long lower facial height (Fig. 6-121).

Osteotomy

A lower buccal sulcus incision is made with subperiosteal dissection performed to the inferior margin of the mandible. Two parallel osteotomies are made horizontally 4 mm below the mental foramen. With a small right-angle saw, the lateral osteotomy is performed bilaterally. The U-shaped bone can be removed and the caudal segment is fixed to the cephalic segment using rigid fixation. An oval burr with a guard is used to smooth the step deformity following the osteotomies on the inferior mandibular margin (Fig. 6-121).

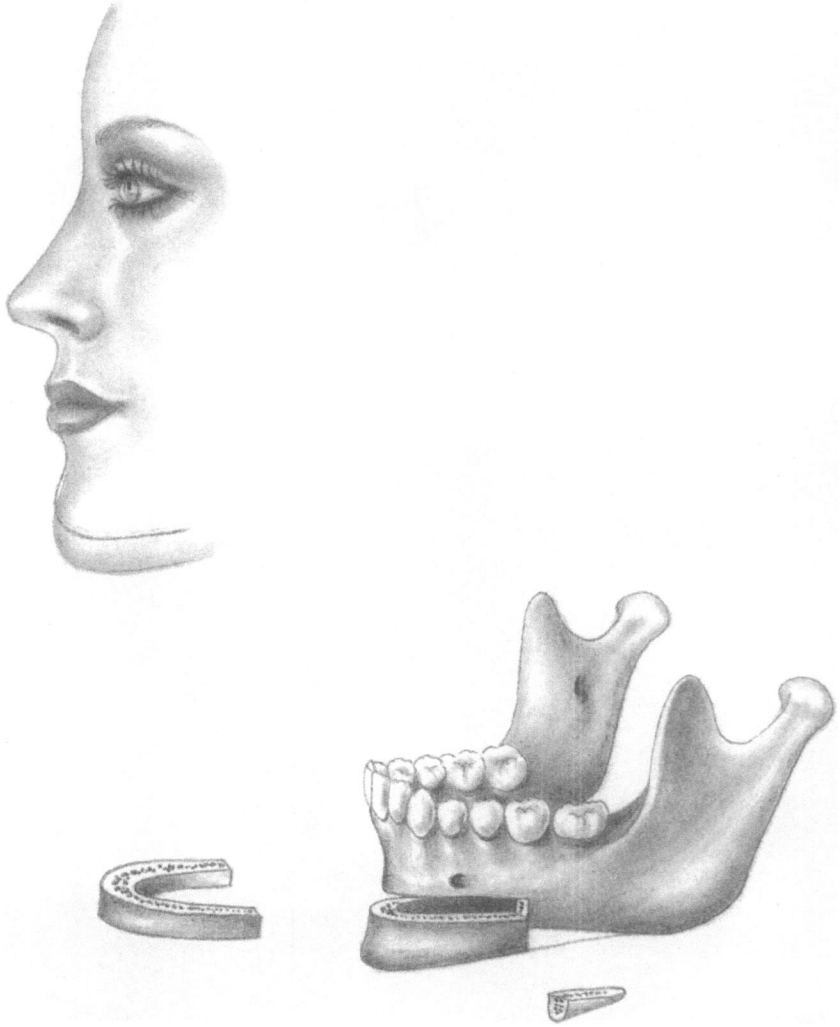

Figure 6–121

Preoperative Evaluation

This patient has a horizontal microgenia. The occlusal relationship is normal (Fig. 6-122).

Osteotomy

The exposure is achieved using a lower buccal sulcus incision. Using an oscillating saw, a horizontal osteotomy is performed 6 mm below the dental apices. A right-angle saw is used to cut the lateral portion of the chin bilaterally. The segment is advanced to the new position and the bone graft is inserted into the gaps. Finally, rigid fixation is employed (Fig. 6-122).

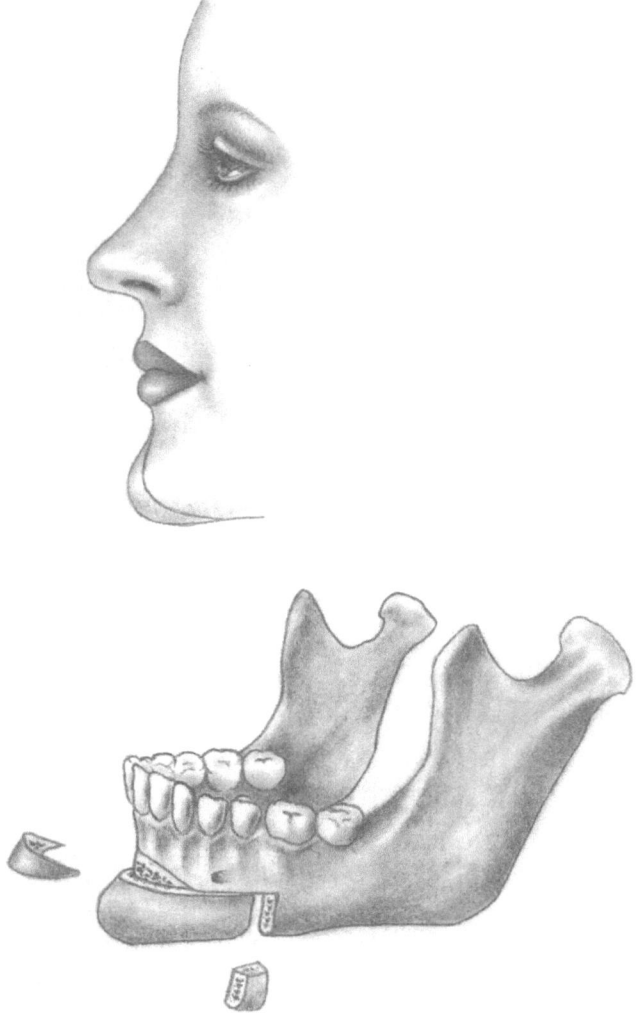

Figure 6–122

Preoperative Evaluation

This patient has an asymmetric chin with a vertical excess of the lower face. The chin point is displaced to the left side. There is no problem with the occlusion (Fig. 6-123).

Osteotomy

A lower buccal sulcus incision is made. The subperiosteal dissection is performed around the incision. Two osteotomies are made asymmetrically according to the preoperative design. A wedge-shaped bone is removed from the left side. Care must be taken to place the cephalic osteotomy at least 6 mm below the dental apices. The caudal segment is fixed to the cephalic segment using rigid fixation (Fig. 6-123).

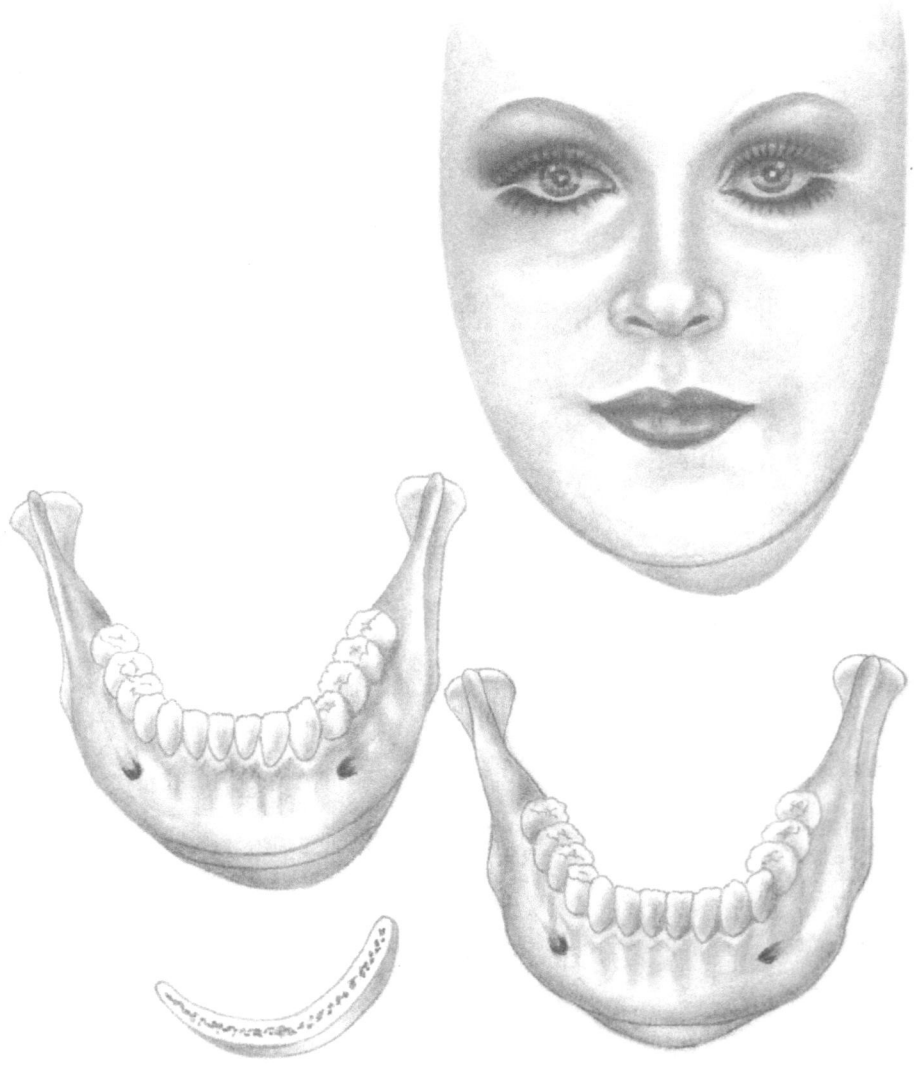

Figure 6–123

Preoperative Evaluation

The patient has a horizontal excess of the chin (Fig. 6-124).

Osteotomy

The incision is made on the lower buccal sulcus and the periosteum is elevated off the mental surface. An oval burr is used to reduce the bone on one side. After the predesigned reduction is done, the procedure is performed on the contralateral side. The wound is closed in two layers. The periosteum must be fixed in order to prevent a chin ptosis or "witch's chin" deformity (Fig. 6-124).

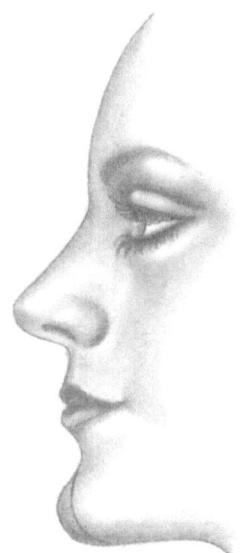

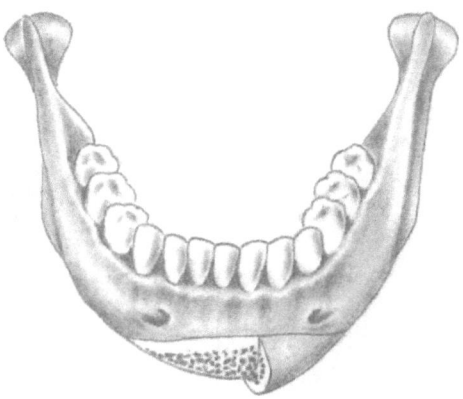

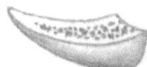

Figure 6–124

Preoperative Evaluation

On frontal view, the patient demonstrates a pointed chin due to the deficiency of the lateral mandibular margin bilaterally (Fig. 6-125).

Osteotomy

The bone graft can be harvested from the cranium. Using a rasp, the bone graft is contoured to the predesign shape. The lower buccal sulcus incision is made bilaterally and subperiosteal dissection is performed down to the inferior mandibular margin. The bone graft is inserted into the subperiosteal pocket and two screws are used for the fixation. Care must be taken not to damage the mental nerve (Fig. 6-125).

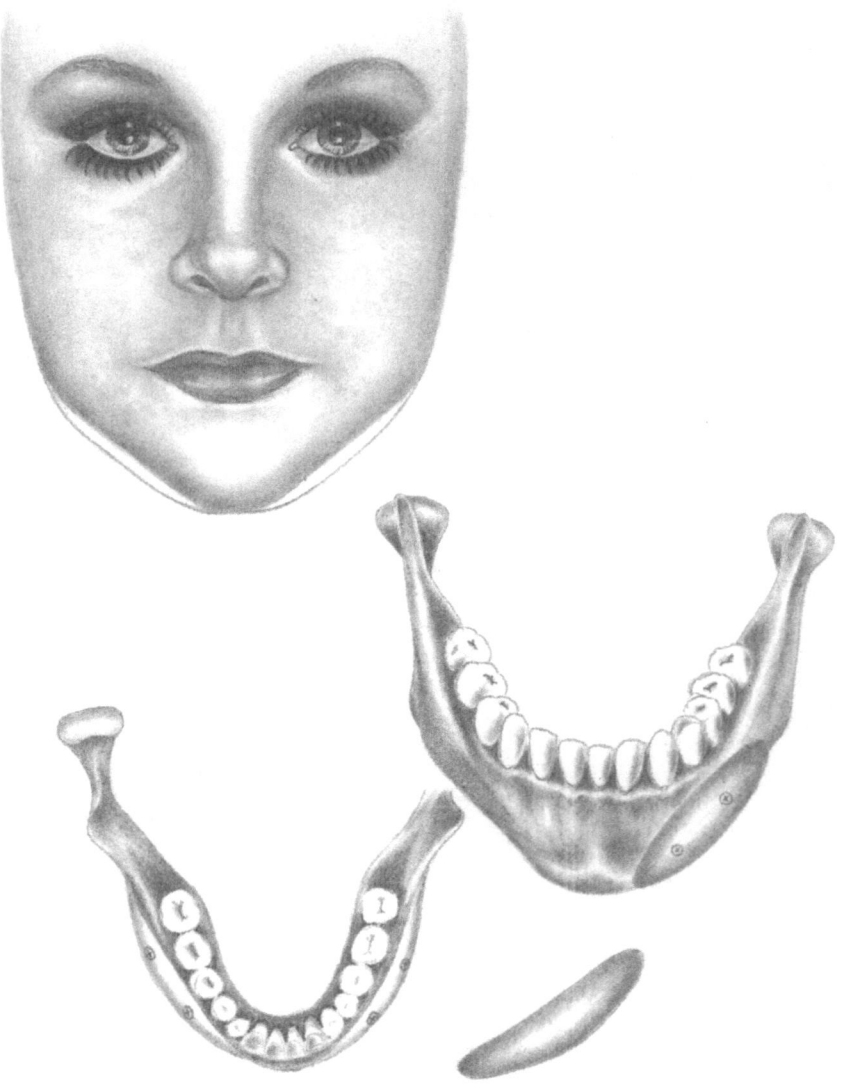

Figure 6–125

Preoperative Evaluation

The front view of the patient demonstrates excess of the mandibular margin bilaterally, which creates the sense of a short face (Fig. 6-126).

Osteotomy

The lower buccal sulcus incision is made bilaterally and the periosteum is elevated down to the lateral inferior roll of the mandible. A reciprocating saw or an oval burr is used to reduce the excessive bone bilaterally. Overcorrection should be avoided. Care must be taken to prevent an asymmetric deformity (Fig. 6-126).

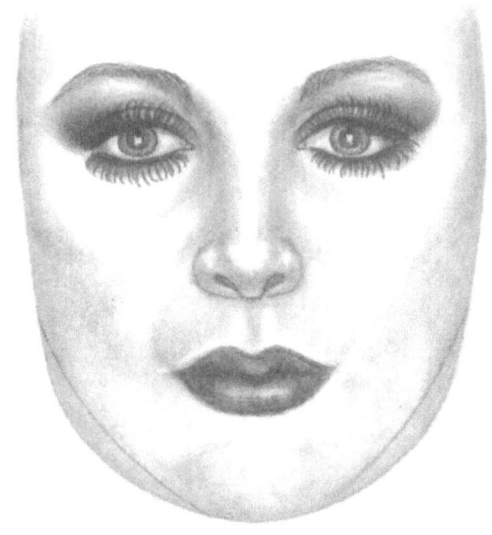

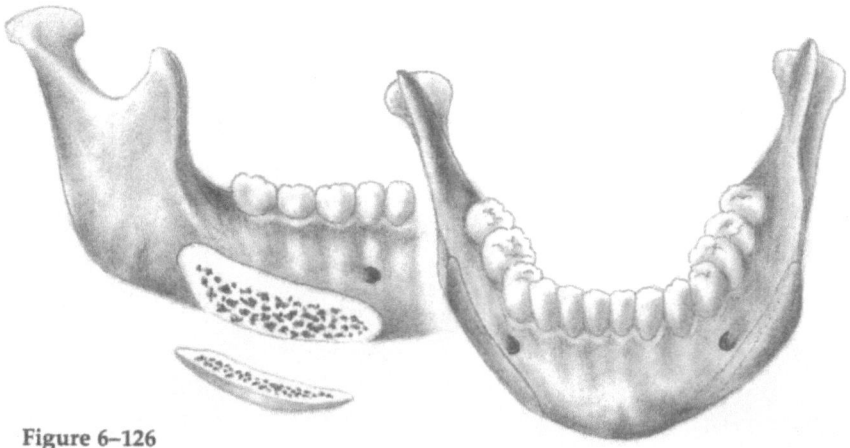

Figure 6–126

Preoperative Evaluation

On lateral view, the patient has a deficiency of the mandibular angle. However, the frontal view demonstrates the bimandibular angle is ideal (Fig. 6-127).

Osteotomy

A posterior buccal mucosal incision is made and the periosteum is elevated off of the superior lateral surface of the ascending ramus. A sagittal osteotomy is made on the area of the mandibular angle and the segment is moved posteriorly. Two screws are placed with a right-angle screwdriver for fixation. The procedure is performed bilaterally. A right-angle oscillating saw is used to trim the posterior rim of the segment (Fig. 6-127).

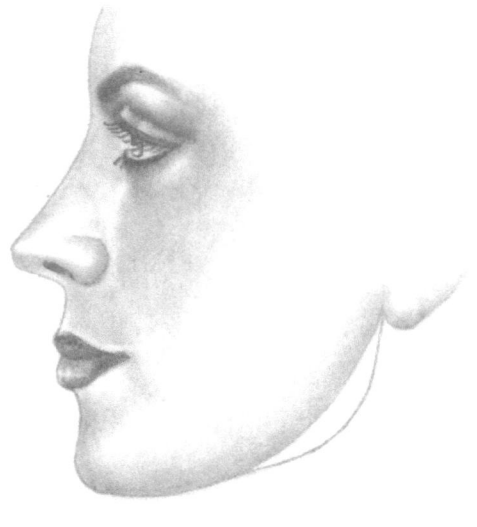

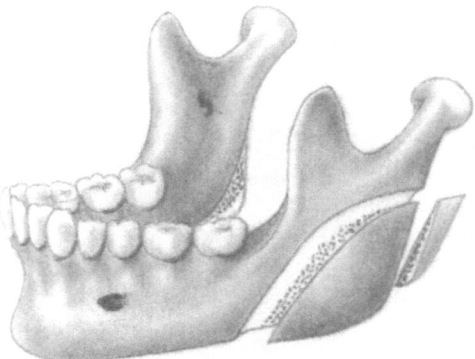

Figure 6–127

Preoperative Evaluation

The patient has a narrow bimandibular angle on frontal view and a deficiency of the mandibular angle on lateral view (Fig. 6-128).

Osteotomy

The bone graft is harvested from the cranium and contoured. Via a posterior buccal mucosal incision, the anterior border of the mandibular ascending ramus is exposed and subperiosteal dissection is made superior to the masseter insertion. With a reciprocating saw, a sagittal osteotomy is made on the lateral angle area down to the inferior border of the mandible. The bone graft, wider posteriorly than anteriorly and wider inferiorly than superiorly, is inserted. Two screws are used for rigid fixation (Fig. 6-128).

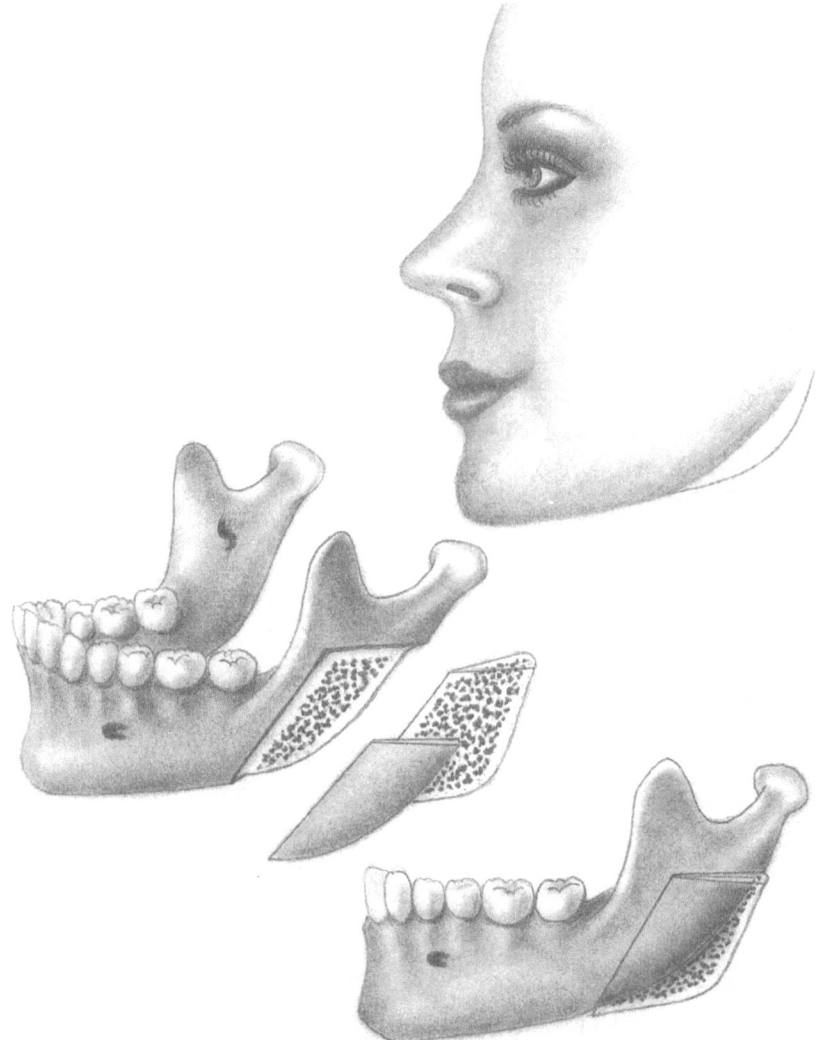

Figure 6–128

Preoperative Evaluation

On lateral view, this female patient has a square mandibular angle, creating a more masculine appearance. Usually, a posterior reduction of the mandibular angle is requested (Fig. 6-129).

Osteotomy

The posterior buccal mucosal incision is used and subperiosteal dissection is made on the lateral ramus. An oscillating saw with a shorter right-angle blade and a long shaft is used to perform the posterior reduction. The symmetry can be obtained with a right-angle burr. Drains and ice packs are applied postoperatively for one to two days (Fig. 6-129).

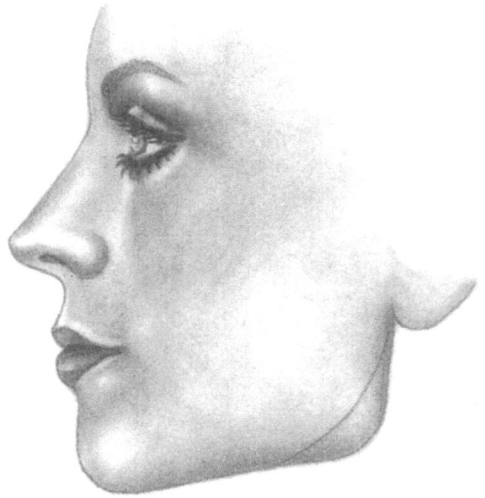

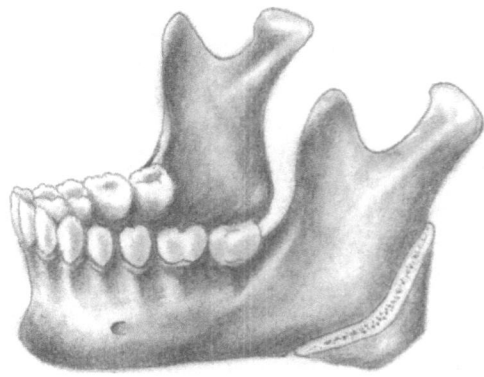

Figure 6–129

Preoperative Evaluation

This patient has a wide face at the level of the mandibular angle. A radiograph demonstrates an extraversion of the mandibular angle. Benign masseteric hypertrophy is not present (Fig. 6-130).

Osteotomy

The posterior buccal sulcus mucosal incision is made with subperiosteal dissection performed on the lateral ramus. With a right-angle burr, an osteotomy is made around the extraverted mandibular angle. The osteotomy penetrates into three-quarters of the thickness of the bone. A greenstick fracture is made along the osteotomy and, using a right-angle screwdriver, rigid fixation is applied. The procedure is repeated bilaterally, and asymmetry should be avoided (Fig. 6-130).

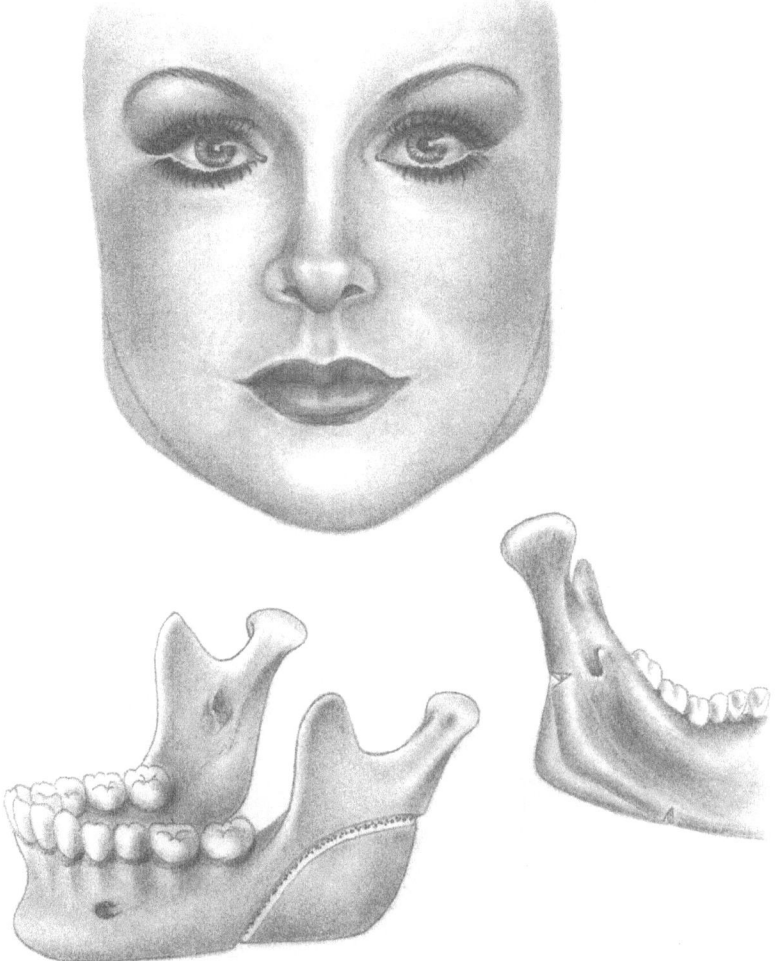

Figure 6–130

Preoperative Evaluation

The patient has a wide bimandibular angle. The posteroanterior radiograph shows the thickened bone as well as benign masseteric hypertrophy (Fig. 6-131).

Osteotomy

A posterior buccal fat pad mucosal incision is made and the periosteum is separated from the lateral ramus to the masseteric insertion. With a retractor, the anterior border of the masseter is exposed. A sagittal osteotomy is made on the medial aspect of the masseter and the lateral aspect of the mandibular angle and the segment is removed. Care must be taken not to damage the posterior and inferior mandibular structures of importance. The procedure is performed bilaterally. It is important to check for symmetry before closing the soft tissues (Fig. 6-131).

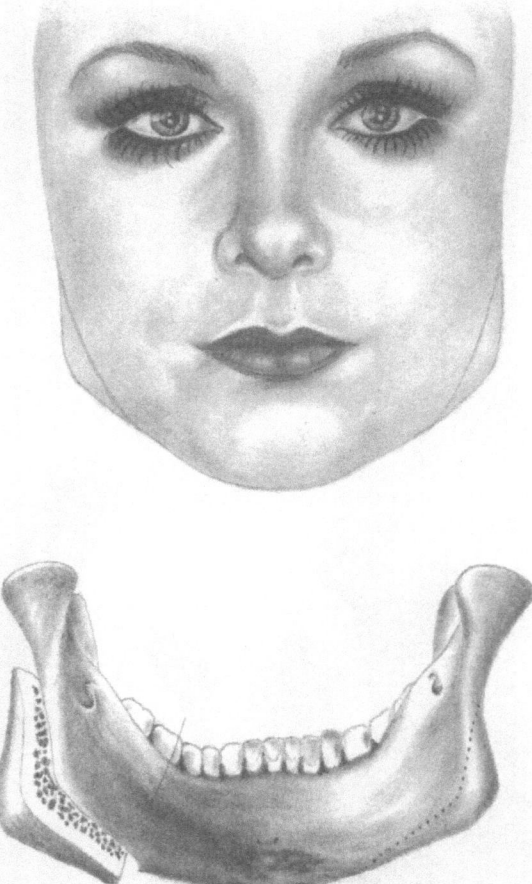

Figure 6–131

Preoperative Evaluation

The patient has a wide lower face. There is an extraversion of the mandibular angle, but the benign masseteric hypertrophy is absent (Fig. 6-132).

Osteotomy

A posterior mandibular angle incision is made and the periosteum is elevated from the medial aspect of the mandibular angle. Using a right-angle burr, an osteotomy is performed around the extraverted mandibular angle. The osteotomy penetrates three-quarters of the thickness of the bone. A greenstick fracture is made medially along the cut and rigid fixation is employed. Care must be taken not to damage the facial nerves. Before closing the wound, symmetry must be checked (Fig. 6-132).

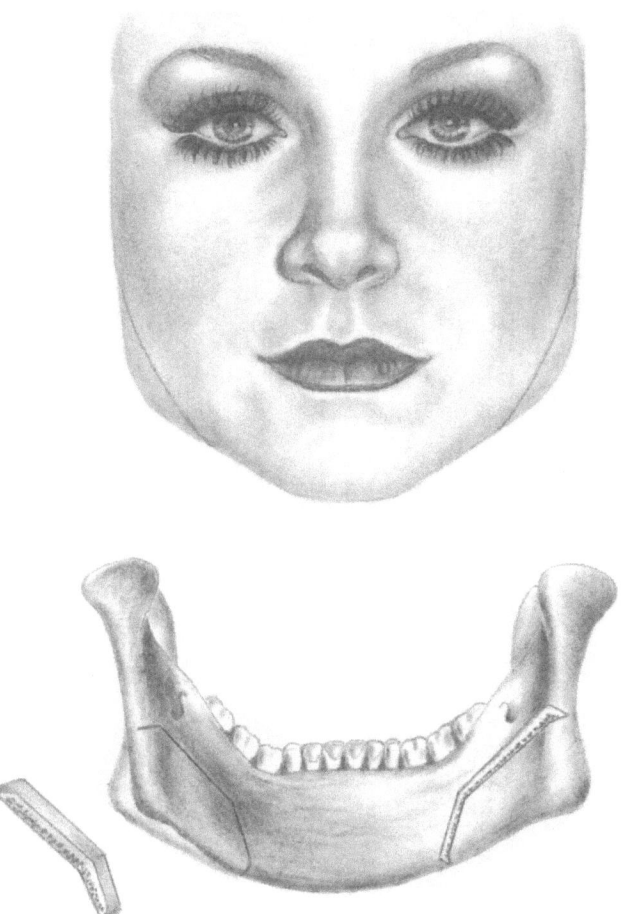

Figure 6–132

Preoperative Evaluation

On frontal view, the patient has a square chin, which is considered a masculine characteristic (Fig. 6-133).

Osteotomy

A lower buccal sulcus incision is made and the periosteum is elevated from the mental surface. With an oval burr, the reduction is performed bilaterally. Overcorrection should be avoided. Care must be taken to prevent an asymmetric deformity (Fig. 6-133).

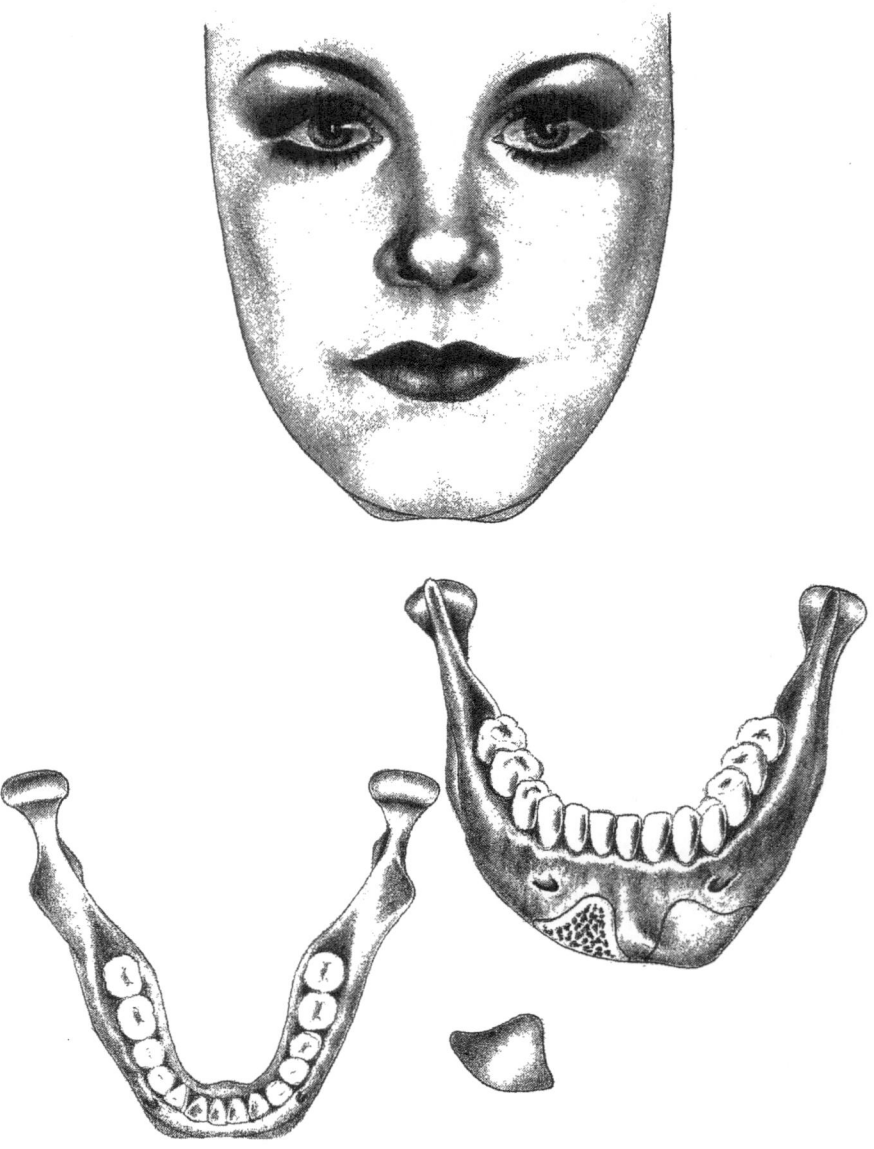

Figure 6–133

Preoperative Evaluation

On frontal view, the patient has an asymmetric chin, which is displaced to the left side, but the vertical height of the lower face is ideal. The patient has a normal occlusion (Fig. 6-134).

Osteotomy

A lower buccal sulcus incision is made for the exposure and subperiosteal dissection is performed along the incision. With a reciprocating saw, the osteotomy is made horizontally 6 mm below the dental apices. The caudal segment is moved to the right side. The mental apex is placed on the midline and rigid fixation employed. Finally, an oval burr is used to trim and smooth the lateral aspects (Fig. 6-134).

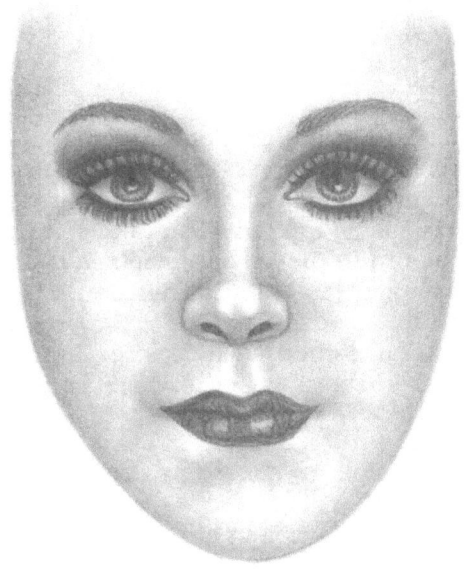

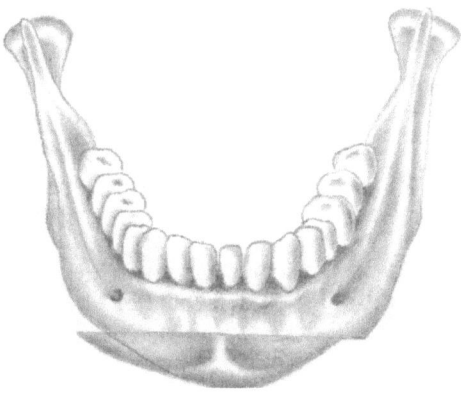

Figure 6–134

7

Osteotomy Fixation

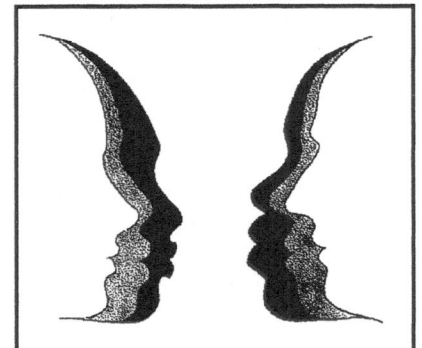

Of great importance to the execution of craniofacial osteotomies is the technology of bone fixation. While some osteotomies are self-stabilizing and require minimal fixation, the majority require a very firm method of stabilizing their position until sufficient bone healing has occurred. As a result, the advancements in the design and fabrication of fixation implants has paralleled that of osteotomies and now provides a wide array of devices for every conceivable application. Potential bone fixation methods include wire ligatures, metallic plates and screws, and resorbable polymer plates and screws.

Wire Osteosynthesis

Stainless steel wire ligatures are a time-proven method of approximating bone segments. Titanium ligatures are available from some manufacturers, but their handling and twisting properties are unfavorable. While wire ligatures are effective at opposing bone edges, they poorly resist rotational movements and are subject to deformation (lengthening) of the knotted wire loop. Therefore, their use should be limited to osteotomy sites that have been designed to be ''self-locking'' or those exposed to minimal deforming forces.

The use of wire ligatures is a simple technique but frequently is done improperly, which can result in decreased loop and knot strength. Twisting of the wire may be done with either a hemostat (28 gauge, .012″ or 30 gauge, .010″) or a wire twister (26 gauge, .016″) and is best done with a twist maneuver executed parallel to the bone surface under continuous tension (pulling). This tightens the wire and places the bone edges under better compression while creating an evenly twisted knot with less risk of breaking (Fig. 7-1, Fig. 7-2). Despite their popularity, other loop (e.g., figure-of-eight) and knot configurations have not been shown to be biomechanically

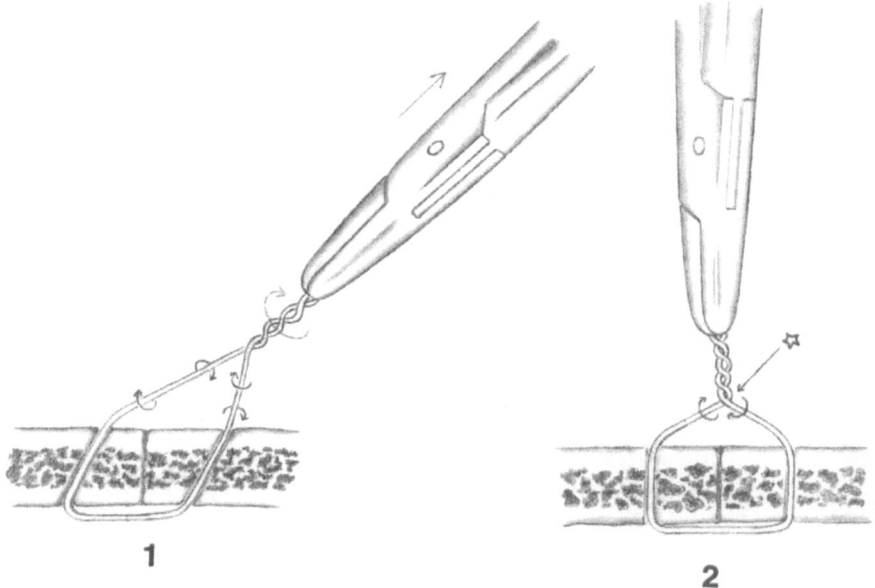

Figure 7-1 1. Correct tightening technique; 2. improper tightening technique.

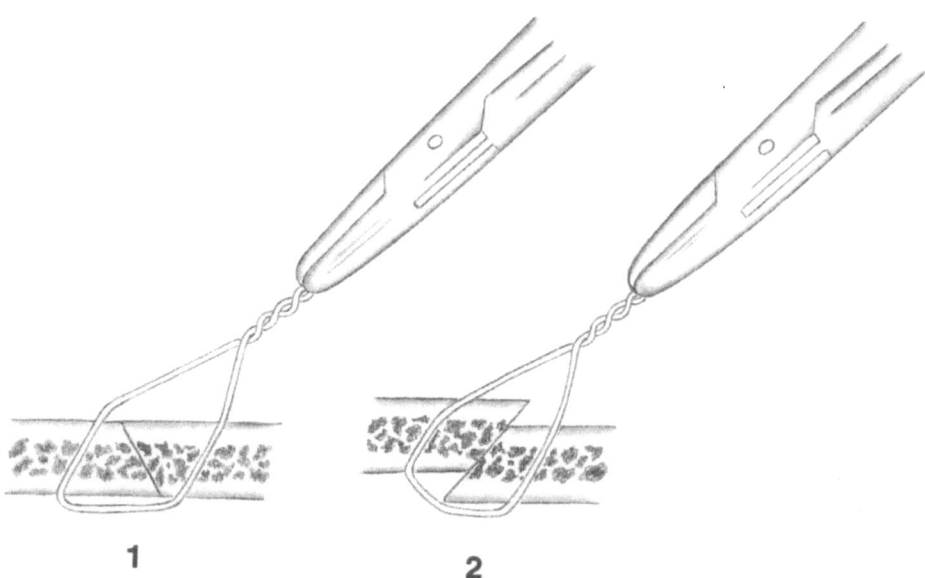

Figure 7-2 1. Correct pulling direction; 2. improper pulling direction.

superior to the simple loop and symmetrical twist adjacent single wire loops are to useful.

Metal Fixation

Current plates and screws are made of either titanium or Vitallium (cobalt-chromium-molybdenum) depending upon the manufacturer. The differences in the physical characteristics of these two metals are of no practical significance in the low biomechanical needs of the craniofacial skeleton, and either material provides excellent fixation. Their use, however, should not be interchangeable amongst the various available sets and manufacturers. Due to the risks of ionic interactions, which lead to corrosion and potential release of toxins into the local tissues, plates and screws of differing metals should not be mixed (i.e., plates from one set should not be used with screws from another system).

Size/Selection

Plates and screws now come in a diverse size ranges, which are primarily determined by bone thickness and extent of exposure to destabilizing forces at the implantation site. They have been historically referred to as miniplates (2.0 mm) or microplates (1.0–1.5 mm) based on the thickness of the plates and width of the screws used, but the recent proliferation in suppliers and manufacturing capabilities has resulted in procedure-specific devices, making this binary classification overly simplistic. While limited biomechanical and engineering data are available to justify the optimum choice of fixation size to osteotomy site, extensive clinical experience confirms the efficacy of the following choices in which all plates are noncompressive and all screws are self-tapping (Table 7-1). The profile of the plate selected is usually only a concern around the orbit and nose, which have a thinner soft tissue cover. Occasionally, secondary removal of the metal devices is necessary in these areas due to palpability or uncomfortable thermal sensations. The thickness of the bone determines the security of engagement of the self-tapping screw. In thin

Table 7-1   Plates and Screws Application

Bone Site	Plate Size (Thickness)	Screw Size (Diameter)
Forehead	0.7–1.2 mm	2.0–2.7 mm
Orbit	0.5–1.0 mm	1.0–1.5 mm
Zygoma	0.5–0.7 mm	1.0–1.5 mm
Maxilla	0.7–1.2 mm	1.5–2.0 mm
Mandible	0.7–1.2 mm	2.0–2.7 mm

bone (<2 mm), microscrews (0.8–1.0 mm) hold better due to a tighter thread pitch. In thicker bone (e.g., calvarium, fronto-zygomatic-facial area), however, the microscrews have a propensity to break while being tightened and a larger diameter screw would be more secure.

Placement Techniques

The placing of a screw through a plate not only secures the plate to the bone but provides the third (vertical) vector for a truly three-dimensional form of fixation between bone segments. The backbone of this system is the integrity of screw placement. A predrilled hole in the bone corresponds to the shaft width of the screw. Wobbling or angling of the drill or overheating due to lack of irrigation results in an asymmetric or widened drill hole, which will require a rescue screw (0.2–0.3 mm wider diameter) for good engagement. The screw is then secured into the hole by the sharp, self-tapping threads that cut into the bone as it is placed and tightened (Fig. 7-3). Some self-tapping screws have flutes at the tips to permit bone debris to escape

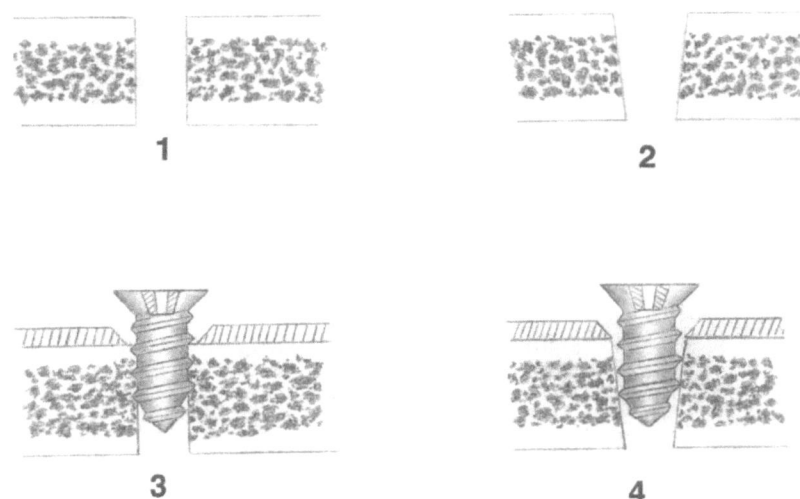

Figure 7-3 1. Proper drill hole; 2. widened drill hole; 3. good thread engagement; 4. poor thread engagement.

as they are placed while other self-tapping screws do not. With the typically "short" length screws used in nonmandibular craniofacial bone (5–9 mm), the lack of a cutting flute has little significance. While pretapping the screw hole is one method of screw placement, there is no biomechanical advantage over self-tapping screws, particularly in the thinner bones of the midface and orbit. Therefore, self-tapping screws are far more popular and simpler to insert due to the elimination of the tapping step.

The use of a lag screw(s) for overlapping bone fragments or for onlay graft fixation is a useful technique in that it results in axial compression between segments. This decreases the amount of micromotion between bone edges and increases the rate of healing. The screw is placed so that the threads do not engage the first segment (glide hole) but tighten securely into the second segment (engagement hole). This requires the use of two differently sized drills, the second of which is equal to or wider than the screw to be used and is only passed through the first segment (Fig. 7-4).

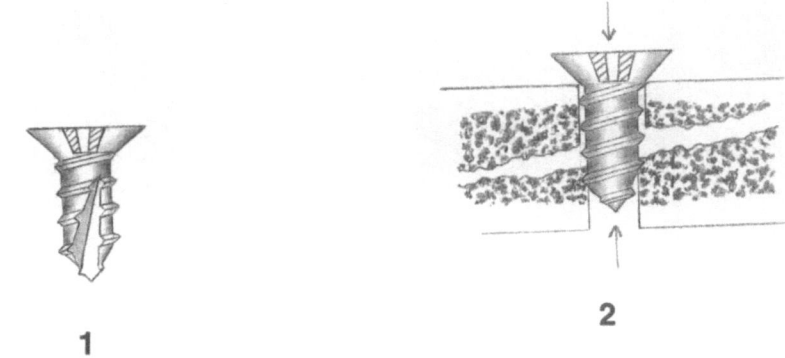

Figure 7-4 1. Self-tapping screw; 2. axial compressive fixation.

All plates used for craniofacial osteotomies are neutral (noncompression). Compression plates are very useful in the trauma patient where realignment of bone contours with good fragment contact is achieved. Osteotomies, however, have bony stepoffs and a mismatch of edges by the design of the cuts and direction of bony movements and so are usually not amenable to the compression principle. Plates of 1.2 mm or less thickness are easy to bend and apply and operative time is not usually saved by the use of templates. Typical plating patterns are illustrated (Fig. 7-5).

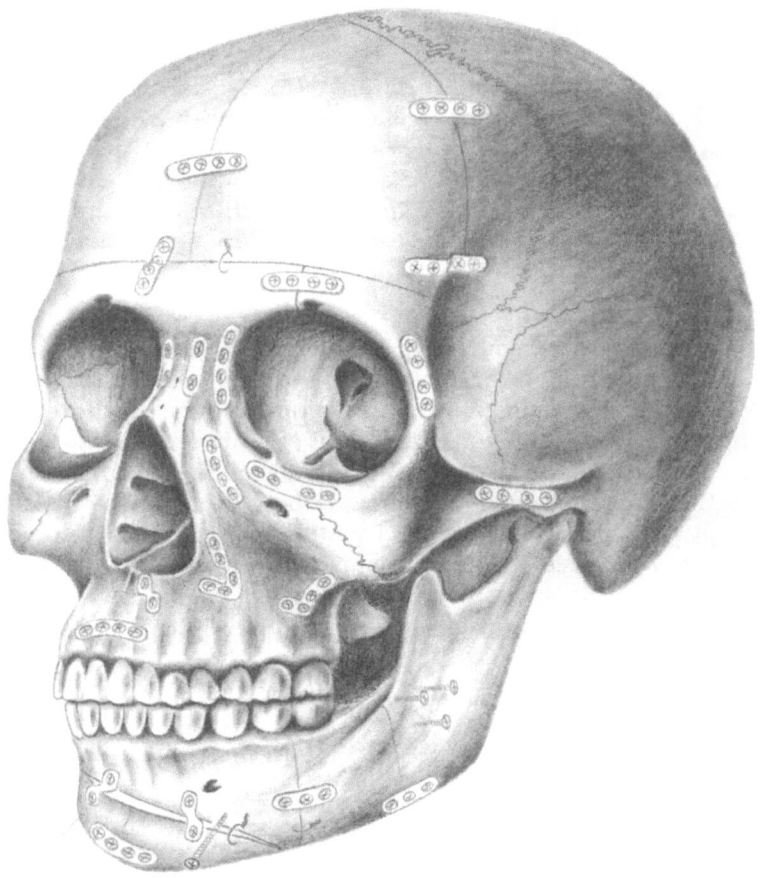

Figure 7-5 Typical plating patterns.

Resorbable Fixation

Unlike metal implants, polymer materials offer the possibility of post-operative device resorption after bone healing has occurred. This would eliminate the potential for device-related complications and the need for their secondary removal. Despite the number of available resorbable polymers (e.g., polylactic acid, polyglycolic acid, polydioxanone), none have been used successfully in humans for craniofacial fixation to date as a monopolymer. The need for sufficient device strength to be maintained in order to allow bone healing to occur while allowing complete device degradation to proceed in a timely fashion without eliciting a foreign-body reaction indicates the need for copolymeric devices. This approach combines the different physical properties of individual polymers to produce a more optimal fixation device.

As polymers are structurally different from metal, their clinical application requires numerous modifications to be successful. Our development and clinical experience with copolymeric (polylactic/polyglycolic acid) fixation in pediatric craniofacial and maxillofacial trauma surgery has permitted insight into these differences. They may be summarized as device design and device application.

Plate Design

The current approach with metal devices is to decrease the volume of metal and miniaturize the devices as much as possible to decrease their postoperative palpability while maintaining the needed strength for bone segment stability. As polymers are inherently weaker materials, mimicry of metal designs would result in insufficient plate strengths. This deficiency is overcome by increasing plate material through greater widths (e.g., 4 : 1 width-height ratio). As such, the approach with polymers is to maximize the amount of material while still permitting the device to be easily applied. As the devices resorb, the "extra" material is irrelevant in terms of long-term postoperative results (Fig. 7-6).

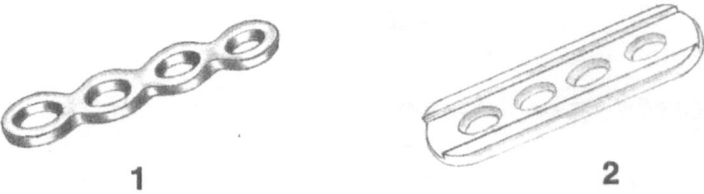

Figure 7-6 1. Traditional metal design; 2. railed resorbable design.

Screw Design

The use of polymers in small fixation devices necessitate a very basic change in screw design. Buttress threads, rather than the self-tapping V-shaped threads of metal screws, must be used to acquire the strength needed to maintain engagement in the bone and prevent screw pull-out and plate loosening (Fig. 7-7).

Plate Application

Polymers are inherently stiffer and less flexible than metals and therefore require thermal manipulation (increasing the polymer's temperature above its glass transition temperature to induce malleability) to induce exact plate-to-bone contact. Many such methods have been proposed but none to date have an easy and safe method of application. We currently use a small, hand-sized heat pack containing an inexpensive chemical compound that when mixed with water results in a sustained heat release exceeding 70°C for 15–20 minutes. This provides a self-contained system onto which the plates are applied, which immediately makes them quite soft (with up to 10 seconds of working time) and allows digital molding to the bone site. This has proven to be a faster method of plate adaptation than that which one experiences with metal hardware.

Screw Application

The change in screw design to a buttress thread necessitates the additional step of pretapping. A pilot hole is initially drilled and then a hand-held tap is used to cut the threads. The screw is then inserted

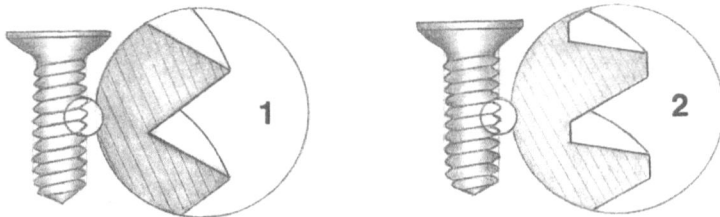

Figure 7-7 1. Metal V-shaped thread design (self-tapping); 2. resorbable buttress thread design (pretapping).

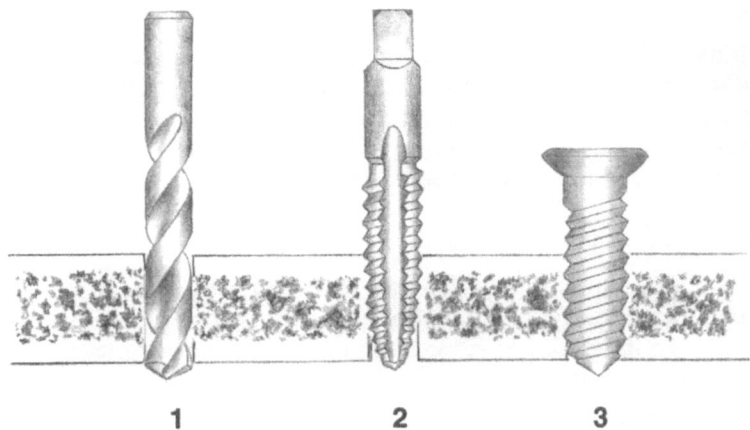

Figure 7-8 1. Drilling of pilot hole (drill diameter = core diameter of screw); 2. tapping to cut screw threads; 3. screw insertion.

until flush with the plate (Fig. 7-8). Currently, screws smaller than 1.5 mm cannot be manufactured with sufficient biomechanical strength to be clinically useful (Table 7-2).

Table 7-2 Screw Placement Protocol

Pilot Hole (Diameter)	Tap (Diameter)	Screw (Diameter)
1.1 mm	1.5 mm	1.5 mm polymeric screw
1.5 mm	2.0 mm	2.0 mm polymeric screw

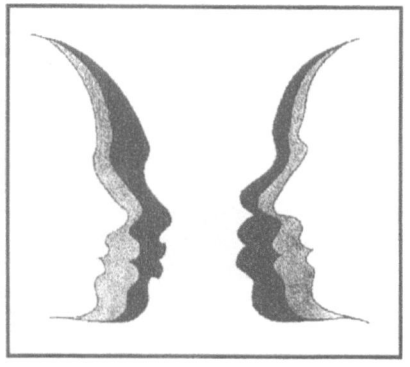

8

Complications

Due to the complex structure of the craniofacial area and the concentration of important organs, aesthetic craniofacial surgery bears relatively higher risks and more complications than other surgeries. For the purpose of reference, we categorize in the following sections the possible problems and complications in aesthetic craniofacial surgery according to the area of operation.

Cranium

1. Dura mater torn and leakage of cerebrospinal fluid
2. Superior sagittal sinus torn and mass bleeding
3. Brain bruising and swelling resulting from overretraction of brain during operation
4. Olfactory bulb damage
5. Subdural hematoma
6. Intracranial infection and meningitis
7. Avascular necrosis of skull
8. Skull surface irregularities and asymmetry
9. Over- or undercorrection of the abnormality
10. Palpable and dislodged fixation materials
11. Baldness and scar alopecia of the scalp

Orbit

1. Corneal abrasion
2. Diplopia and strabismus
3. Reduction of visual fields and loss of vision
4. Supraorbital nerve damage
5. Oculomotorius and trochlear damage

6. Ptosis
7. Lacrimal gland damage
8. Nasolacrimal duct damage and obstruction
9. Palpebrum ectropion and entropion
10. Frontal sinus problems
11. Intraorbital infection
12. Retro-ocular hematoma
13. Over- or undercorrection of the abnormality
14. Step-abnormal of orbital edge
15. Antimongoloid sloping of the palpebral fissure

Maxillae

1. Mass retro-pharynges hematoma
2. Damage to the great palatine vessels and nerves
3. Infraorbital nerve damage
4. Damage to frontal branch of the facial nerve
5. Perforation and deviation of nasal septum
6. Nosebleed
7. Oral-nasal sinus problems
8. Maxillary sinus problems
9. Avascular necrosis of maxilla
10. Over- or undercorrection
11. Malocclusion
12. Velopharyngeal incompetence and speech problems
13. Devitalized and luxated teeth
14. Exposure of teeth roots
15. Gum recession
16. Asymmetry
17. Serious swelling and airway obstruction
18. Gap inflammation
19. Pressure temporalis (extruded) and chewing problems after greenstick fracture of zygoma

Mandible

1. Damage to inferior alveolar nerves
2. Gap inflammation
3. Damage to mandibular glands
4. Damage to carotid sheath
5. Avascular necrosis of mandible
6. Lower lip paralysis
7. Devitalized and luxated teeth
8. Exposure of teeth roots
9. Gum recession
10. Chin ptosis
11. Irregularities and step-abnormal of infra-edge of mandible
12. Over- or undercorrection
13. Asymmetry

14. Malocclusion
15. Tongue-swallowing and airway obstruction
16. Jaw ankylosis after intermaxillary ligature fixation

Other Complications

1. Psychological change and postoperative psychosis
2. Transmitted diseases, such as AIDS and hepatitis, caused by blood transfusion
3. Laryngomucosa swelling and airway obstruction resulting from repeated intubation
4. Heart and lung function problems due to inappropriate volume replacement of blood lost or fluid and electrolyte disturbance
5. Donor site morbidity
6. Hypertrophic scarring and keloids
7. Wound and bone infection
8. Bone graft resorption

Measures to Reduce Complications

1. Have an overall understanding of the patient's psychological situation and free the patient's mind of misgivings.
2. Perform an overall physical examination and evaluation to eliminate contraindications.
3. Administer a mass dose of antibiotic preoperatively, intraoperatively and postoperatively.
4. Perform atraumatic and meticulous operative technique.
5. Apply controlled hypotension and hypothermia anesthesia to reduce blood loss and catabolism.
6. Separate cranial cavity operation from oral or nasal cavity operations.
7. Make a precise evaluation of the patient's face and the patient's expectation of the operative result.
8. Avoid entering paranasal sinuses and repair any perforation before the operation is finished.
9. Irrigate the operative field with antibiotic solution frequently.
10. Design ingenious osteotomies to reduce the incisions and the area undermined and peeled.
11. Apply stable fixation methods after bone movement.
12. Improve performance and increase accuracy to reduce operative time.
13. Maintain close observation postoperative and intensive care.

9

Future Developments

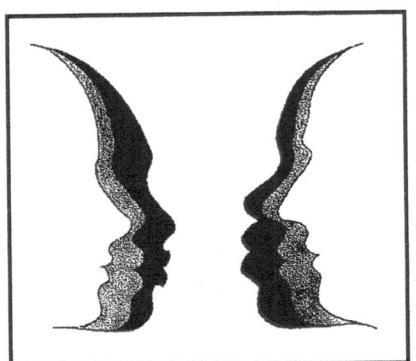

For I dipped into the future
Far as the human eye could see
Saw the vision of the world
And all the wonder that would be
Tennyson

Craniofacial surgery is derived from the surgical experience of World War I, the contributions of European maxillofacial surgeons between the two world wars, and, most importantly, the pioneering work of Paul Tessier. Like all surgical milestones, Tessier's contributions were based on research—countless cadaveric dissections of the craniofacial skeleton.

Craniofacial surgeons have been adept at promoting and conducting research, as well as at rapidly integrating disparate technological developments into the mainstream practice of craniofacial surgery. For example, many of the advances during the last 25 years have been resulted from developments in the fields of digital imaging and materials sciences. In addition, the surgeon has benefited from health care improvements in pediatric anesthesia and the development of intensive care units.

Progress usually occurs in periodic bursts, with relatively quiet intervening periods. Consequently, it is difficult to predict accurately future developments and trends in craniofacial surgery. Progress will most likely occur as a result of developments in the following areas: 1) digital imaging; 2) biomaterials technology; 3) bone biology; 4) soft tissue healing; 5) minimalization surgery; and 6) clinical and molecular genetics.

Digital Imaging

Computerized tomography (CT) and digital imaging have already had a tremendous impact on all fields of medicine. The ability to break a complex image down into digital data has largely removed the constraints imposed by the oversimplified two-dimensional format of conventional radiographs. Standard radiographs have been limited by the superimposition of all structures between the x-ray beam and the film. Moreover, the nonparallel nature of the beam can cause problems with magnification. There is often difficulty with standardization of technique and comparability of films, especially with asymmetric craniofacial anomalies (e.g., cephalogram dependency on external auditory canal rod standardization in the craniofacial microsomia patient with microtia).

CT and magnetic resonance imaging (MRI) scans circumvent the problems inherent in conventional radiographs as described above. Anatomic structures are clearly delineated, as the confusing superimposition of images is essentially avoided. Furthermore, the images are standardized to a given scale, as the distance between the x-ray source, the patient, and the detector are fixed and invariant. These modalities allow a more precise delineation of the nature of the pathologic anatomy. For example, individual aspects of the calvarium may be viewed free from the distortion of superimposed structures. The anatomy can be viewed from many different perspectives (axial, coronal, etc.). As the software has progressed, the latticework of data points to be reconstructed in a three-dimensional format, allowing the software to provide highlighting and shadowing of surfaces to provide a three-dimensional image on two dimensional imaging film.

Therefore, the first impact of digital imaging is that it has helped the craniofacial surgeon define the pathology in the individual patient with greater accuracy. One is reminded of Tessier's global search for museum skull specimens in an effort to study the anatomic details of various craniofacial anomalies; contemporary three-dimensional CT scanning can provide a library of stereolithographic models of any anomalous craniofacial skeleton.

The second, and perhaps more important impact of digital imaging and computerized tomography on craniofacial surgery is that it provides the surgeon with an important tool that can be used longitudinally to: characterize how a clinical problem may change with the critical variables of growth and the elapse of time; analyze the effect of surgical intervention on the clinical problem; and study the effect of surgical intervention with time and growth. Because all data points are standardized, a comparison of CT scans at different time points provides significant data. In a preliminary fashion, CT scans have been used to construct normative standards as well as inventories of the characteristics of complex deformities. It is only recently that CT scans have been used to characterize the effect of surgical intervention on clinical problems and to provide a standardized, reproducible format for data exchange between various craniofacial centers. The ability to quantitate change will allow more accurate definition of the efficacy of various treatment approaches and, as a consequence, lead to a refinement of techniques. However, one must recognize that a significant stumbling block to the accumulation of such data is parental and societal concerns about the cumulative radiation exposure to the patient.

In the immediate future, there will undoubtedly be improvements in hardware, such as with the spiral CT scanners that are now becoming widely available, allowing faster scanning times. These faster scan times allow narrower scan slice widths to be routinely used. Therefore, instead of a routine 3- or 5-mm scan slice width, widths of 1 mm may be routinely used. As the number of data points increases in the latticework, the resolution improves dramatically. As the number of hard data points is increased, the approximations and rounding performed by software becomes more precise. Increased data provide increased resolution and improvements in multiplane reformatting. This allows a given data set to be rotated on various axes and output in more usable formats without sacrificing anatomic accuracy. The cost of imaging and digital data storage should also continue to decrease.

Digital data can also be employed in the operating room to allow precise localization and translocation of skeletal landmarks during surgical procedure. The initial generation of intraoperative aids is currently available. These devices allow the surgeon to visualize the exact position of a special instrument (wand) in sagittal, coronal, and axial planes of digital images in real time. As software and hardware continue to improve during the next decade, these initial instruments may allow precise movement (translocation) of skeletal segments in three dimensions and allow realistic execution of precise preoperative plans. Moreover, the development of such technology will result in a trend away from large skeletal (monobloc) movements toward multisegment advancements in order to simulate more closely the normal anatomy. Robotic operative surgery is currently being practiced by the orthopedic surgeons to core the femur to produce a recipient site for a precise fit of a hip prosthesis in order to obviate the need for glue with attendant implant interface fractures.

Advances in digital imaging and data storage will allow an accumulation of experience and exchange of data among surgeons and international craniofacial treatment centers leading more importantly to a critical interpretation and assessment of data. No longer dependent on before and after kodachrome slides of variable quality for evaluation of treatment protocols, the clinician will have the opportunity to refine existing techniques and, more importantly, develop new treatment approaches. These digital images can also be an extremely powerful tool in teaching, from the level of the medical student to the fully trained craniofacial surgeon.

Biomaterials Technology

In the future, the advances in biomaterials should continue. There exists the distinct possibility of the development of the ideal biomaterial, which should theoretically be totally resorbable and be replaced by bone before resorption is complete.

At the current time biomaterials fall into three main categories: metallics, polymers, and ceramics. There has been a dramatic increase in the use of metallics in the past decade, primarily adopting and adapting the successful experiences of the Swiss A.O. group (Arbeitsgemeinschaft für Osteosynthesefragen) and others, to the repair of craniofacial structures. Improvement in plate fabrication with titanium and cobalt/chromium alloys, and a reduction in sizes have made their use practical and routine in the craniofacial region. Although such benefits as ease of application, improved fixation, and stability, and avoidance of intermaxillary fixation are strong considerations, enthusiasm should be tempered by the cost of the plating systems and other concerns. In the infant, the effect of implantable devices on subsequent craniofacial growth and the migration of metallic plates and screws with penetration of the dura during cranial vault remodeling have been discussed.

A recent alternative to metallic systems are absorbable plating systems. The combination of poly(lactic acid)/poly(glycolic acid) (PLA/PGA) as copolymers provides favorable stability and resorption characteristics. By varying the concentration of lactide and glycolide monomers within the composition of the polymeric chain, this copolymer marries the strength and resorption characteristics of each individual material. The copolymer shows excellent tissue compatibility and is broken down primarily by hydrolysis. In animal models the copolymer does appear to be extremely well tolerated, without evidence of a significant foreign body reaction. This copolymer ratio has been used for years as a synthetic, resorbable suture material and has an established track record in routine clinical use. In the limited number of secondary operations performed on craniofacial cases, there has been complete plate resorption by six months. Furthermore, we have not performed any secondary operation for complications related to resorbable plate use, such as irritation, inflammation, or non-union. This system, or other polymers and copolymers, may provide an alternative to permanently implantable devices in the craniofacial region.

As a separate application, other polymers and compounds have continued to be developed for augmentation of the facial skeleton. Previously the main goal was to develop substances that were totally unreactive and inert; current research goals are to produce polymers that allow implant integration by enhancing the interface between the implant and the osseous recipient site.

The best example of successful bioactive interfaces are the ceramics. Although extremely hard and brittle, they can provide an effective material for augmentation of the facial skeleton in selected applications. The materials have been developed to the point where hydroxyapatite (calcium phosphate derivatives of coral) readily allows ingrowth of native tissues, synthesis of osteoid and bone in the pores of the hydroxyapatite, and effective bonding between the newly synthesized bone and the implant. In addition, Inote, a ceramic coralline derivative of calcium carbonate, may allow complete replacement by bone, therefore satisfying one of the theoretical requirements of an ideal bone substitute.

In a more global perspective, the long-term future for biomaterials is less predictable. As the number of regulatory restraints increases, the development of new materials and approaches may be constrained. In an era of health care reform, financial constraints represent another consideration. One can speculate whether the development costs, the costs of meeting increased regulatory testing, the costs of defensive strategies in an overly litigious society, and the costs of marketing are merited in the new health care environment?

Bone Biology

It is, perhaps, in the elucidation of the natural processes of bone synthesis, remodeling, and healing that the greatest advances in craniofacial surgery can be realized. Such insights, gained from the application of the principles of molecular biology, would allow the surgeon to manipulate the normal and pathologic skeletal environment.

Osteoinduction is the biologic phenomenon of inducing bone formation in a biologic milieu. After the initial insight provided by Dr. Charles Huggins, additional understanding of this phenomenon has been provided by Dr. Marshall Urist and Dr. A. Hari Reddi. Through the efforts of these investigators and their earlier work with demineralized bone preparations, the isolation of the bone morphogenetic proteins (BMP) has come to fruition.

BMP belongs to the transforming growth factor beta (TGF-β) superfamily of growth factors. At present, there is considerable interest in understanding the role of these growth factors in terms of their interplay with organic and inorganic matrices. The BMP's have already been used to prefabricate bone segments with specific shapes and characteristics, albeit in animals with lower metabolic rates than primates. In addition, they have been applied to carriers to replace full-thickness defects in canine mandibles. The ability to manipulate osteoinduction in the human could represent an enormous step in replacing bony (inlay) defects and in onlaying the deficient craniofacial skeleton without the need for the harvesting of autogenous bone grafts.

The other side of the problem, and equally important, is to understand how to limit bone formation and inhibit growth in a controlled fashion. In the neonate and infant, bone formation and bone healing occur at an accelerated pace. A delayed union or nonunion in fracture management in the infant is uncommon. In the early days of infant craniofacial surgery, it was recognized that postsurgical cranial defects heal rapidly. Consequently, the concept of a critical-sized defect has little meaning. In a laboratory study of cranial defects, Dr. Craig Hobar and associates demonstrated that immature dura possesses unique osteogenic properties, which are lost as the animal matures.

The mechanism of successful inhibition of bone formation in the normal calvarial suture has yet to be elucidated. This would be an extremely important finding, since it essentially provides a model for successful, focal inhibition of bone synthesis and the maintenance of cranial suture patency. Through the application of the techniques of molecular biology, this mechanism should be completely elucidated.

Soft Tissue Healing

Most of the emphasis and advances in craniofacial surgery have centered on the reconstruction of the craniofacial skeleton. Yet, the limitations in completely successful craniofacial surgery rehabilitation are often apparent in the overlying soft tissue envelope, manifest by deficient and scarred tissue. In other words, there remains a significant soft tissue problem in craniofacial surgery. Microvascular free flaps have been successfully employed to address the overlying soft tissue deficiency by augmenting the underlying skeleton to restore facial contours in such conditions as craniofacial microsomia and hemifacial atrophy (Romberg's syndrome). Other extensions of this technique include microvascular free composite flaps that contain vascularized bone as part of the microsurgical reconstruction.

Recent work in fetal wound healing has demonstrated that the fetal environment is unique in that wounding of soft tissue results in a type of healing which is free of gross and microscopic evidence of scarring. If this environment and/or factors can be successfully applied in the mature surgical patient, it would be an enormous advance eliminating the scar sequelae of surgical incisions and enhancing the final surgical result.

Minimalization of Surgery

The manipulation of osseous healing, as exploited clinically with the distraction of the mandible and other components of the craniofacial skeleton, represents a forward leap into the minimalization of craniofacial surgery. It was Gavril Ilizarov of Russia who demonstrated the clinical efficacy of the technique with his reconstruction of various deformities of the long bones of the lower extremities, which are of endochondral origin. Dr. Joseph McCarthy and his colleagues subsequently demonstrated the feasibility and application of the technique in the membranous bones of the facial skeleton. Their work, and that of others, supported Ilizarov's law of tension stress that ''living tissues, when subjected to slow steady traction become metabolically activated in both the biosynthetic and proliferative pathways, a phenomenon dependent upon both vascularity and functional use''. The technique is essentially based on the creation of an osteotomy/corticotomy and application of an external fixator with a screw driven mechanism, followed by progressive bone lengthening at the osteotomy site at a rate of a millimeter per day. This results in the creation of substantial regenerate bone at the osteotomy site.

The advantage of distraction osteogenesis is the superior quality of the bone that is generated. Unlike traditional bone grafts, there is little evidence of clinical resorption or relapse. In the craniofacial region, where the bones are thinner and the regional blood supply is superior, the application of the technique has less morbidity than in the lower extremity. More importantly, there is not only the gradual expansion of bone but also of the associated soft tissues, thus also improving the functional matrix and reducing the relapse rate after mandibular or maxillary advancements.

With the refinement in techniques and the development of new distraction devices, the technique has also been applied experimentally to the cranial vault, the orbit, the zygoma, and the midface. The technique offers the advantage of reduced operating time, shortening hospital stays, and obviating the need for bone grafts and blood transfusions. The endoscope can be used to perform various craniofacial osteotomies with limited dissection and blood loss. In the future, the combination of endoscopy and distraction may represent the ultimate step in the minimalization of craniofacial surgery.

Clinical and Molecular Genetics

Significant advances and increased understanding in molecular genetics have resulted as part of the international effort to map the genome (Human Genome Project). The most impressive findings have been the mapping of various genetic loci and the identification of mutant genes for several craniofacial syndromes including Crouzon, Apert, Pfeiffer, and Jackson–Weiss syndromes. It has been demonstrated in these craniofacial synostosis syndromes that the mutations lie in the gene family of receptors to fibroblast growth factors (FGF-R). It is speculated that different types of mutations within each syndrome account for the observed variability in phenotypic expression.

The opportunity for prenatal genetic counseling, and even gene engineering, are enormous. Probably no area of research will have as profound effects on the future development of craniofacial surgery as will the disciplines of clinical and molecular genetics.

Predicting the future is extremely difficult, if not treacherous. We do know, however, that the rate of advances will be even more accelerated in the future, and no one can predict where the next rush of insight will occur. As has been said in the past, "the only constant in life is change" and craniofacial surgeons must be prepared not only to adapt to change but to take advantage of it. They must work with their colleagues since advances in the laboratory will have enormous effects on the evolution of this surgical discipline. Craniofacial surgeons must not only support and encourage research but, in an era of constrained resources, they should also be staunch advocates for continued support of research activities for the benefit of their patents, and also staunch advocates for the optimal clinical care of their patients.

Recommended Reading

Complex Craniofacial Problems. New York: Churchill Livingstone. Dufresne, Craig R. 1992.

Complications in Head and Neck Surgery. St. Louis: C.V. Mosby. Eisele, David W. 1993.

Changing the Body. Baltimore: Williams & Wilkins. Goin, John M. 1981.

Genioplasty. Boston/Toronto/London: Little, Brown and Company. Guyuron, Bahman 1993.

Atlas of Craniomaxillofacial Surgery. St. Louis: C.V. Mosby. Jackson, Ian T. 1981.

Techniques in Aesthetic Craniofacial Surgery. Philadelphia: Lippincott. Salyer, Kenneth E. 1988.

Plastic Surgery of the Facial Skeleton. Boston/Toronto: Little, Brown and Company. Wolfe, S. Anthony 1989.

Rigid Fixation of Craniomaxillofacial Skeleton. Boston: Butterworth-Heinemann. Yaremchuk, Michael J. 1992.

Aesthetic Contouring of the Craniofacial Skeleton. Boston/Toronto: Little, Brown and Company. Ousterhout, Douglas K. 1991.

Index

The letter f following a page number indicates a figure.